Advance Praise for *Star*

"Emily Boller's story is of enormous importance and will help many people. This is the only book on eating disorders that grasps the critical significance of the Standard American Diet as a contributing cause and that correctly identifies nutritional density as an essential aspect of recovery. *Starved to Obesity* is foundational to true recovery and turns recovery into something attainable and natural rather than a perpetual struggle. Beautifully, magnificently done! ...Emily has such a critical message and is the perfect messenger for a new era in medicine!"

— Jeffrey Rediger, M.D., MDiv, Faculty, Harvard Medical School, Medical Director of Adult Psychiatric and Community Programs at McLean Southeast, McLean Hospital–Affiliate of Harvard Medical School; Chief of Behavioral Medicine at Good Samaritan Medical Center

---

"*Starved to Obesity* gives us a compelling insight into the fundamental reasons behind food addiction and binge eating. Growing up with a mother whose love language was cooking and baking, to the terrible tragedy of losing her son; food became Emily's refuge. Ironically, turning to food (*the right kind*) was the solution to attaining her optimal weight. *Starved to Obesity* offers a science-supported, practical guide to finding a healthy relationship with food. It's well researched and wide reaching. If you struggle with your weight and want to learn from someone who has 'been there, done that,' this book is for you."

— Dr. David Friedman, Syndicated TV/Radio Health Expert, #1 International Bestselling Author of *Food Sanity: How to Eat in a World of Fads and Fiction*

"Emily Boller draws upon her personal journey of tragedy to triumph to create a clear, hope-filled pathway to healing and wholeness. If you, a friend, or loved one struggle with dieting, emotional eating, weight loss, or health challenges, *Starved to Obesity* can change your life. It is a beacon of hope and a north star pointing the way to freedom."

— Scott Stoll, M.D., *Alive! A Physician's Biblical and Scientific Guide to Nutrition*, Co-Founder and Chairman of the Plantrician Project, Author, Speaker, Olympian

———————

"In *Starved to Obesity,* Emily Boller bravely shares her inspiring journey out of despair after stunning life tragedies left her drained of direction and trapped in a fortress of fat from out-of-control eating. Candidly, lovingly, with nutritional pearls aplenty, Emily shares her hard-won wisdom and practical advice for overcoming adversity and making delicious, health-promoting dishes that can help you transform the direction of your life to one of health and rich enjoyment of every day and every meal. I will recommend this wonderful book to all of my patients struggling with weight, food addictions and emotional challenges of many kinds. Thank you, Emily, for *Starved to Obesity*—it is a gift to us all."

— Michael Klaper, M.D., Nutrition-based Medicine Expert, Author, Speaker

———————

"We are facing an epidemic of obesity and Type 2 diabetes with its acute, chronic, debilitating, deadly diseases. Fast food and sugars are horribly addictive. This book completely describes the problem and gives a solution. A great book! I would recommend it to everyone."

— Rudy Kachmann, M.D., Neurosurgeon, Author of Fifteen Wellness Books, TV and Radio Wellness Authority

---

"Emily Boller is an inspiration to everyone who knows her. As a formerly obese mother of five children, she is living proof that you, too, can finally overcome your battle with food. *Starved to Obesity* will not only teach you how to do it, but it will also leave you feeling Emily's warmth and understanding that you are not alone. It's time to be set free!"

— Sarah Taylor, MBA, MS, *Vegan in 30 Days, Vegetarian to Vegan*

"Emily Boller's writings and presentations are engaging, authentic, and applicable for today's culture. Her insights are the result of experiencing devastating loss and triumphal victory along her journey towards a healthy lifestyle."

— Ken Hood, Wellness Director at James River Church in Springfield, Mo.

"Emily Boller is a great example of identifying and gaining victory over some monumental issues in her life. She has embodied the theme of 'Not Somehow, But Triumphantly.'"

— Carl Sovine, Ph.D., Licensed Marriage and Family Therapist

"I loved *Starved to Obesity*! It was raw, liberating, and empowering...offering hope and inspiration for anyone seeking to embrace a healthy lifestyle."

— Kristin Misner Meier, MSPT, Wife, Devoted Mother of Three

"The truth in this life-giving book will set you free. Thank you, Emily, for your vulnerability, wisdom, and grace."

— Carol Doscher, President and CEO, Graceworks Inc., New York City

---

"Emily Boller has faced her own eating challenges with unflinching honesty, unfailing open-mindedness, and unflagging persistence. Learning from her journey has equipped me with important guidance and tools for my own journey."

— The Rev. Dr. Susan Gilbert Zencka, Frame Memorial Presbyterian Church in Stevens Point, Wis.

STARVED TO
OBESITY

**MY JOURNEY OUT OF FOOD ADDICTION
AND HOW YOU CAN ESCAPE IT TOO!**

Emily Boller

Foreword by **Joel Fuhrman, M.D.**

Post Hill
PRESS

A POST HILL PRESS BOOK
ISBN: 978-1-64293-051-1
ISBN (eBook): 978-1-64293-052-8

Starved to Obesity:
My Journey Out of Food Addiction and How You Can Escape It Too!
© 2019 by Emily Boller
All Rights Reserved

Cover art by Cody Corcoran
Cover photos by Ruth Yaroslaski

All Scriptures taken from the Holy Bible, New International Version ®, NIV ®, Copyright © 1973, 1978, 1984, 2011 by Biblica, Inc. ™ Used by permission of Zondervan. All rights reserved worldwide. www.zondervan.com The "NIV" and "New International Version" are trademarks registered in the United States Patent and Trademark Office by Biblica, Inc. ™

Post Hill Press
New York • Nashville
posthillpress.com

Published in the United States of America

*To my husband, Kurt, who has graciously learned
to love me unconditionally and support me wholeheartedly
in sickness and in health.*

Disclaimer

The following pages are my unique story of food addiction. I am not a physician, psychologist, or theologian. This book is not intended as a replacement for medical, psychological, or spiritual advice and care. A health care professional should be consulted if you are on medication or if there are symptoms that may require medical or psychological attention.

CONTENTS

FOREWORD

I first met a smiling, healthy-looking Emily Boller in 2009 in an airport after she had lost more than a hundred pounds following my Nutritarian diet-style. We had never met before, and she did not consult me about her weight and health issues. She also had done it without any local friends or family to support her, and she had significant obstacles thrust in her path, yet she persevered. Emily had read my book, *Eat to Live,* and applied the information on her own with fierce determination. I had seen her photos and corresponded with her by email, and she was at the airport to be a success story on a television interview I was doing.

She kept journalistic documentation of her transformation with great photos and verbal accounts of the transformation that took place, as she essentially became a different person.

Since then, Emily has spoken at my Health Getaway events, has written wonderful, uplifting and insightful blog articles, and has interviewed scores of others who have also transformed their lives. She has learned a lot and is now a scholar in this field of health transformations. I am not only grateful for her sharing her impactful health makeover in my books and television appearances, but also grateful for her insight and motivation through her writings that she has given to so many thousands of members at DrFuhrman.com and on my blogs.

Losing more than one hundred pounds in one year can be hard, but it can be made so much easier when you have the right information at your fingertips to help you navigate the obstacles in your path. The secret to success is to develop fluency in these advances in nutritional science and understanding of food addiction that forms the body of knowledge supporting a Nutritarian diet. A Nutritarian diet is a style of eating that focuses on healthy foods that prolong the human life span. However, the same anti-cancer and longevity-promoting diet-style is also the most effective way to achieve reversal of chronic diseases (such as diabetes and high blood pressure) and the attainment of a healthy weight that you can maintain for the rest of your life. For successful adoption and full enjoyment of this lifestyle, education and training is essential.

Emily has been there and has triumphed in spite of incredible obstacles and personal tragedy. She has managed to collect gifts of wisdom that she has compiled and earned along the way, gifts that she now bestows on you. The gifts are given with the hopeful expectation that you will benefit in some way from her experience, insight, and knowledge.

I am grateful for the opportunity I have been given to be useful in some way to so many people, too, but both Emily and I know it is not just about the number of people; it is about the profound and lifesaving effects that have occurred and can occur for many who are struggling to be set free from the mind-controlling effects of processed foods and the deadly American diet that leads to incredible human suffering and kills people needlessly every minute. I hope you will study her words and continue your

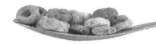

quest for knowledge, as that is truly the only road to great health and lasting happiness.

Emily has demonstrated her remarkable desire to extend herself to help others in need over and over, asking nothing in return. She sets a standard of ethics and compassion to emulate, and I am proud to be her friend.

— Joel Fuhrman, M.D.
   Board-certified family physician specializing in
      nutritional medicine
   President, Nutritional Research Foundation
   Six-time *New York Times* bestselling author

AUTHOR'S NOTE

I will freely admit my life had spiraled out of control into the perilous abyss of food addiction and binge eating. The oppression eventually consumed my every waking moment as it slowly dominated my life, changing the very person I was until I didn't even recognize myself anymore. By that, I mean physically, yes, but also emotionally and psychologically.

Why in the world would I divulge this dark secret? Why would I expose my intensely personal life to you, a complete stranger?

It is not my intent to share my story merely for the sake of creating another weight loss memoir that will wind up collecting dust on a shelf.

No, I have written this book because I wholeheartedly wish there had been a book such as this when I was a kid. It would have been helpful to me and to those in my circle of influence: parents, teachers, coaches, clergy, youth workers, camp counselors, physicians, friends, and my future husband. It would have been priceless information that could have possibly saved me and my then-and-future family many years of needless pain and suffering.

My husband and I were on a walk recently, and I was lamenting about the fact that when I was in my twenties there wasn't a book that I had access to on the topic of food addiction. In the midst of my pity party, he suggested, "Maybe it is because you had to experience it yourself so that you could understand

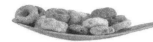

others' pain and suffering in order to help them." And maybe he was right.

I *do* understand the pain of those suffering with food addiction.

And I care.

Whoever you are, whether you are struggling to hold life together in the midst of addiction or you're a concerned person wanting to know how to help someone you care about, my story is for you. Let me come alongside you and offer my experience, guidance, hope, and motivation.

As you read the following pages, please don't be in a hurry. Take time to assimilate every chapter. They are simple, but powerful.

May this book bring freedom to you and those you care about and want to help.

Here's to great health to all.

— Emily Boller

"I freed a thousand slaves.
I could have freed a thousand more
if only they knew they were slaves."

–Unknown[1]

1   "Unknown Quotes." BrainyQuote.com. Xplore Inc, 2018,
    accessed May 5, 2018. https://www.brainyquote.com/quotes/
    unknown_388682.

CHAPTER 1

A NEW ENDING

"Emily, the police are here, and Daniel is dead."

It was like any other day until I heard my husband's voice on the other end of the phone telling me those chilling words.

That day in 2012, our twenty-one-year-old son had died by suicide.

Once the initial shock wore off, I sank into a suffocating depression. It also ignited a latent binge eating disorder.

Experiencing the symptoms of complicated grief caused me to realize how much I had suffered from bouts of depression and binge eating for *much* of my life, not just post-tragedy. The family trauma, naturally, took it to a whole new level, but it had been percolating underneath the surface since childhood. Like Robin Williams, I could easily mask my inner angst with a cheery disposition.

My first recollection of the blues and bingeing occurred during the time that my parents were remodeling their old farmhouse in rural Northeast Indiana. I was in sixth grade. I clearly remember getting off the bus, entering the house. Large sheets of black plastic closed off every room and window except a small space, big enough for a table and chairs. It was a major renovation of their kitchen and dining room, and it became a beautiful

Better Homes and Garden project afterward. Walls were knocked out and windows were added to open up space and add natural light, and new cupboards, countertops, light fixtures, and appliances were installed. But the process was dark and suffocating for a kid.

There was no place to go; nothing to do in the house. It was like entering a dark cave for days on end. Looking back, the darkness, boredom, and loneliness inside the house stirred a gloomy depression and addiction that had been lurking within me. I clearly remember eating an entire package of Oreo cookies in one sitting after school one day.

By that time in my life, my sweet tooth was highly developed. Processed baby formula in infancy was little more than artificial junk food laced with corn syrup that later gave way to sugar-sweetened processed cereals and homemade baked goods.

My mother excelled in the culinary arts, and her way of expressing love was through cooking and baking. As a result, she was one of the best pastry chefs around: apple cake and apple crisp, rhubarb crunch, German chocolate cake, butterscotch cake, angel food cake, carrot cake with cream cheese frosting, multiple birthday cakes throughout each year, coffee cake, strawberry shortcake, lemon bars, banana nut bread, chocolate chip cookies, chocolate-covered peanut butter balls, iced Christmas cookies, cheesecake with cherry topping, chocolate fudge, and homemade jams. Her pies with their flaky crusts were renowned: blueberry, cherry, apple, rhubarb, strawberry, pumpkin, and pecan with whipped cream or vanilla ice cream a la mode. Why, she could turn a plain ol' zucchini into a confectionary work of art.

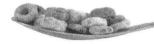

She also sweetened *everything* with sugar: potato salad, coleslaw, deviled eggs, pickled eggs, beets, baked ham, yams, chili, sloppy Joes, peaches, strawberries, stewed apples, even sliced tomatoes. There was also a bowl of sugar on the table to sweeten breakfast cereal each morning. Sugar was a mainstay seasoning in her kitchen.

On top of all that sugar continuously pulsating through my veins, I collectively drank gallons of milk, orange juice, sweetened lemonade, Kool-Aid, and Tang each week, and consumed an excessive amount of Halloween, Christmas, Valentine's Day, and Easter candies throughout the year.

Since there were always plenty of baked goods and sweets lying around, including quarts of ice cream and boxes of Popsicles, Fudgsicles, and Hostess Twinkies in the freezer, I binged regularly. The seeds of a food addiction were planted, and no one seemed to notice or care.

It goes without saying that I became "pleasingly plump" as a result, so I was put on a calorie-restrictive diet in first grade. I was sent to school with a Thermos of chopped lettuce, hard-boiled egg slices, diced ham, and Catalina salad dressing poured over it; plus, half a grapefruit. (By lunchtime, the contents of that Thermos were a lukewarm, soggy mess.) I was also weighed daily, and my weight was recorded on a chart. I got a plus sign if I lost weight, but a "goose egg" if I gained.

As one might expect, the diet didn't work. I didn't lose one pound. Instead, my six-year-old psyche gained an undue pressure to be thin and developed a preoccupation with weight and appearances—and guilt. Additionally, I also developed an abnormal aversion to scales. I especially dreaded them at school when the nurse would weigh everyone for report cards in front of snickering classmates.

Unfortunately, and unbeknownst to anyone, the constant barrage of sugar poisoning on my developing brain, combined with a lack of vital nutrients, was altering the very chemistry and health of it. It didn't stand a chance. The deadly combination was putting my brain at risk and was significantly damaging my body on the cellular level as well...one bite at a time.[2, 3]

The worst part about being overweight in childhood was not the poor health and lethargy per se; nor was it wearing the homemade and unflattering "tent dresses" because normal clothes in the Sears catalogue were out of the question; nor was it needing to put corn starch between my chubby thighs to prevent painful chafing; or even being the last one picked for gym class teams. The worst part was enduring ongoing verbal assaults: Moose, Fatso, Fatty, Porky, "Here, sooey, sooey, sooey.... Here, sooey, sooey, sooey"—the call for pigs at feeding time. One day, I was warned that livestock trucks were coming to take me to the slaughterhouse.

For whatever unfortunate reason, I made the seventh-grade cheerleading squad. I was an anomaly out on the gym floor: the plus-size teen in pigtails wearing a short, homemade, form-fitting

2   Jayanthi Maniam, Margaret Morris, "Sugar may be as damaging to the brain as extreme stress or abuse," *The Conversation,* February 15, 2016, assessed May 3, 2018, https://theconversation.com/sugar-may-be-as-damaging-to-the-brain-as-extreme-stress-or-abuse-53813.

3   Joel Fuhrman, M.D., *Disease-Proof Your Child,* (New York: St. Martin's Press; 2005), 79.

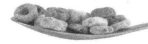

uniform that exposed pudgy legs and rolls of fat. The cruelty of the shouts from the bleachers, especially from the opposing team's fans, cut me to the core. The searing pain and humiliation were unbearable at times.

Teachers, recess aides, parents, coaches, bystanders... *someone* should have intervened to prevent the assaults; however, back in the '60s and '70s, emotional and verbal abuse was acceptable and allowed. Combined with the nonstop sugar overload on my developing brain, all of it was the perfect petri dish for depression and addiction to incubate simultaneously. "Sticks and stones may break my bones, but words will never hurt me" is a lie. A big fat lie.

Many research studies have linked physical and sexual abuse to lasting effects on the brain, but emotional abuse has been relatively overlooked. However, Martin Teicher, director of the Developmental Biopsychiatry Research Program at McLean Hospital and an associate professor of psychiatry at Harvard Medical School, along with three colleagues—Jacqueline Samson, Ann Polcari, and Cynthia McGreenery—did a comparative study of the impact of childhood verbal abuse. They found that "verbal abuse had as great an effect as physical and extrafamilial sexual abuse." Teicher even concluded, "Verbal abuse may have more lasting consequences than other forms of abuse, because it's often more continuous."[4]

---

4   William J. Cromie, "Verbal beatings hurt as much as sexual abuse; Can lead to depression, anxiety, and worse," *Harvard Gazette,* April 26, 2007, assessed May 2, 2018, http://news.harvard.edu/gazette/story/2007/04/verbal-beatings-hurt-as-much-as-sexual-abuse/. Text used by permission of Martin Teicher, M.D., Ph.D.

There was no escape from being overweight in childhood. That Oreo binge in sixth grade was the beginning of a depression-triggered eating disorder.

Bingeing morphed into a panicky desperation to be thin by the time I was in eighth grade in 1975. It was imperative for me to be normal, likable, and to fit into a pair of jeans by high school. It was not merely a desire. It was survival. It was the only way out of the verbal abuse, the discrimination, and the isolation. I severely restricted calories and ate only an orange for lunch at school every day and started running for the first time in my life.

It worked. The pounds melted off, and I entered high school at normal weight. All abuse stopped, and I actually became popular. I made the "pom pom squad" and performed during half-time at home basketball games. I ran the mile in track and won first place in most meets. I had cute clothes to wear and a date for each prom. I was inducted into the National Honor Society and even won the Miss Congeniality Award in the school's Junior Miss Pageant.

However, in the spring of my senior year, I came home from school one day to learn my mom had made arrangements with a doctor for me to be hospitalized for "tests." An eye doctor had called her earlier in the day. He was concerned that I might have diabetes because a recent eye exam had revealed a significant change in my vision.

Mom had just gotten off the phone from the hospital as I walked in the door. They had a bed ready and would be waiting for my arrival. Being the caring mother that she was, she complied

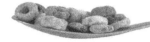

with the professionals' recommendations. She instructed me to pack a change of clothes and a toothbrush.

I thought perhaps I was going for an overnight stay.

I had no clue I would be spending *many* nights there.

I was admitted that afternoon to the fifth floor, the geriatric unit of the hospital. I was never told the reason why I was admitted to that particular floor.

My elderly roommate suffered from diabetes complications. We had nothing in common. In fact, I had nothing in common with anyone on that floor. I didn't even have to wear a hospital gown like everyone else.

I was an active seventeen-year-old missing track practice. It snowballed into missing the entire track season—not to mention senior-year festivities.

Smartphones, iPads, and social networking sites were nonexistent. The isolation suffocated me. I had nothing to do except lie on a sterile bed and wait for more testing.

My room was located at the end of a hallway. Across from it was a metal door to a dimly lit stairwell that no one used. At night, when my roommate was asleep and I knew the nurses wouldn't be checking on me, I would sneak out and run up and down several flights of stairs for more than an hour. The vigorous workout was a part of my mental and emotional survival. It enabled me to release my pent-up anger and counteract the boredom.

The meals delivered to the geriatric floor were less than appetizing: a slab of softened meat or scoop of macaroni and cheese, a slice of white bread, an overcooked vegetable, applesauce or stewed fruit. And the food service workers didn't care when they came to pick up my barely touched tray of leftovers.

In addition to daily urine and blood tests, another test clearly stands out in my mind: my first gynecological exam.

A doctor and his female assistant led me down a dark, abandoned hallway on that geriatric floor. Surplus gurneys lined both sides of it. We stopped at an empty room with an exam table in it.

The doctor instructed me to remove all my clothes and to lie down on the table. He and his assistant repositioned my body and put my feet into metal stirrups.

There was no such thing as searching the internet for information back then. I had no idea what lay ahead.

Neither the doctor nor his assistant explained anything to me. Most likely it was just a rote procedure to them—one of thousands.

As the doctor spread my legs apart, I tensed up. The cold, stainless steel speculum penetrated painfully. In that moment I realized I had no choice but to consent to the unknown.

They both told me to relax—which was impossible—so the assistant held my hips in place while the doctor performed the procedure.

Afterward, I was told to put my clothes back on. The assistant escorted me back to my room in silence.

The worst part of the hospitalization was the day of discharge. I had lost a significant amount of weight since the day I was admitted. The attending physician told me to take all my clothes off and stand in front of my parents. He proceeded to show them every part of my naked and emaciated body. He didn't even possess the decency to drape a sheet over me.

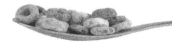

Then he pointed to my breasts and called them "infantile." He told my parents that I would never be able to have children. He spoke to them as if I weren't in the room.

I had no place to hide. I couldn't even cover my private parts with my arms and hands due to the visual examination. The exposure was humiliating as I stood there on display.

The many tests revealed that I did *not* have diabetes. Instead, the doctor sent me home with a diagnosis of a low thyroid level and anorexia nervosa, an eating disorder characterized by weight loss or lack of appropriate weight gain. Back in the late '70s, anorexia was not a relatively well-known affliction like it is today. He instructed my mom to follow up with an internist for my thyroid condition and to make me eat more food—which opened the door for major food battles when I returned home. The strife created ongoing tension, which intensified my loss of appetite.

Unfortunately, I was too weak to be part of the track team—a devastating loss to me.

My chronic self-deprivation of nutrients and calories, combined with my low body weight and mounting inner turmoil, eventually triggered depression. The lack of fat on my body also decreased my capabilities to keep warm, concentrate, and use good judgment.

My periods stopped, my ribs and shoulder blades protruded, I had lost muscle mass in my upper arms and thighs, and my body grew some white, soft downy hair to insulate itself.

I was a mess.

Today, we know much more about the brain, and we recognize it can become injured and/or sick, as with every other organ of the body. But in the late '70s, mental illness had great stigma and shame attached to it. My parents swept the eating disorder diagnosis under the rug and never mentioned it again—even though my emaciated condition was obvious.

Instead, that summer after graduation, I was discreetly sent to live with an older brother and his wife in Wisconsin. At their home, the food battles were nonexistent, and I was able to relax and eat meals in peace. As a result, I gained just enough weight to attend Purdue University in West Lafayette, Indiana that upcoming fall of 1979; otherwise, I wouldn't have had the physical stamina to walk to classes on such a large campus.

Sadly, the pendulum swung back to binge eating. No one knew I was struggling with depression and addiction. I could easily mask my inner turmoil and angst with a gregarious smile and keep the weight off with diet and exercise. Once more, I was popular and usually had a date every weekend.

In the midst of this active eating disorder my freshman year at Purdue, I met a junior named Kurt.

He lived with forty guys in a house named Fairway that was part of the cooperative housing system on campus, and I lived with nearly thirty girls in a house named Twin Pines. It was customary for the male co-op houses to invite the female co-op houses to social activities called "functions." And it was impolite not to show up. Everyone was expected to participate.

Fairway had asked Twin Pines to a roller skating function. I skated with several of the guys that night, but Kurt was the only one who offered to take me home afterward. And I accepted.

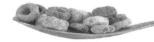

He was unlike any guy I had ever met before. He was polite, and he respected me enough not to force a kiss on me when we arrived back at my house. He simply stated that he had a nice time and would like to see me again. He also added that he would be praying for me.

His kindness endeared my heart to him that night.

We dated the remainder of that academic year. For the summer, he drove to Colorado to work on a dude ranch. Those three months of physical separation drew us even closer, as we exchanged love letters.

When Kurt arrived back to campus after his cowboy adventure, it was obvious to everyone that we were now a couple.

He asked me to marry him soon after Christmas break that year.

I hesitated for a bit, primarily because I was only a sophomore, but also because I knew I had unresolved issues with food.

I confessed to Kurt that I had a "food problem," but he shrugged it off by reassuring me, "Everyone eats an extra piece of cake now and then."

Being in denial of the severity of the problem myself, I wholeheartedly agreed with him. Everyone *does* eat an extra piece of cake now and then...no big deal.

I was just nineteen and my parents had only met Kurt two times. But with their blessing, he proposed to me—and I accepted.

We planned the wedding for the summer after my sophomore year.

I had met his dad one time, and I met his mom two days before the wedding. She had driven her red, sporty MG convertible all the way from California.

(Years later, I learned that my parents didn't think I was ready for such a commitment, but they didn't want to interfere with our plans.)

I had remained slender the entire year of dating and during our engagement, but shortly before the wedding, Kurt commented that I needed to lose a few pounds.

My mind immediately tumbled right back into the pit of unrealistic expectations and pressures to be thin, which was like throwing a lit match into a container of gasoline. I should have postponed the wedding, but love had pulled the shades down on my vision.

I didn't call off the wedding. Instead, on a hot August day in 1981 we exchanged vows in an unairconditioned country church that I had attended throughout my childhood. We honeymooned for several days in Northern Michigan before moving into a scorching cinder block apartment in married student housing at Purdue.

Due to lack of income, I worked at a drugstore near campus while Kurt finished his final semester of undergrad studies. Suddenly, my active social life came to a screeching halt as I managed a mundane, full-time job, grocery shopping, preparing meals and clean-up, thank you notes for the many wedding gifts, and mounting piles of dirty laundry. I had been an athlete in high school; the domestic arts were not my forte. I was totally unprepared for the responsibilities of married life, so I turned to food in order to cope.

As a result, I gained weight. My clothes no longer fit. The minimum wage I received barely covered our basic necessities. We couldn't even afford curtains let alone new clothes.

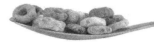

Thankfully, my uniform at the drugstore was an oversized smock that hid the extra pounds. At home, I wore old stretchy sweatpants and t-shirts. However, anxiety consumed me when I ran into friends on campus. The self-imposed shame of the weight gain created an unhealthy obsession to lose it…but I just kept binge eating and gaining instead.

Kurt and I were both very young, and the eating disorder was way more than either of us could understand or handle on our own.

Kurt became verbally abusive in those early years of marriage—an unhealthy behavior he had learned in childhood. He called me such names as Fatso, Frumpola, Pudge, and Slob. My eating disorder escalated as the weight gain and name-calling spiraled out of control.

To escape the ongoing torment and emotional pain, I continued to numb myself with food. For example, I would pour half a box of Grape Nuts into a large bowl. Then I would pour milk over the cereal, just enough to cover it, followed by spoonfuls of sugar. Within minutes of eating it, I would begin to feel drowsy, and then I would fall asleep and not wake up for a couple of hours.

These ongoing bingeing episodes induced "food comas" that enabled me to psychologically escape the undesirable life I felt trapped in at the time and anesthetize the wounds of domestic abuse—not fully realizing that the emotional eating was also contributing to my inner strife and turmoil.

Gradually, babies came along. *So much for the doctor's proclamation to my parents when I was seventeen that I would never have children—I ended up having five children by age thirty-seven!* The food struggles got so bad that I eventually mustered up enough courage to reach out and confide with an older woman. She gathered a few women around me to pray. I was told that I must have trafficked in witchcraft and sorcery since childhood. I was so confused and embarrassed afterward.

Prayer services and church-related activities that I attended—whether large corporate gatherings or in-home Bible studies—served doughnuts, cookies, and the like. Gluttony not only prevailed in these spiritual settings, but it was promoted, and it perpetuated my addiction. The sessions added an additional layer of confusion and complication to my downfall.

I tried every Bible verse and diet imaginable to cast out the supposed demons within, but to no avail. I was trapped in a besetting sin, yet I saw no way out of the misery. I even attempted a forty-day fast amidst cooking for and raising five children and managing the busy household.

On the thirty-third day of drinking only water, I went grocery shopping and nearly passed out in the middle of the store. I suddenly became dizzy as I gorged on the sights and smells of food. I had to sit and call Kurt to come to get me, because I was too weak to finish shopping and make the short drive home. Out of sheer frustration, coupled with being famished, I abruptly ended the fast and succumbed to binge eating all over again. It started with eating buttered popcorn, several apples, a banana, a few slices of whole wheat bread, and lettuce with shredded cheese poured over it—on an empty and shrunken stomach. Afterward, the pain was unbearable, but that didn't deter me from devouring more food.

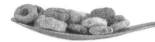

Despair set in, and I felt hopeless. I eventually gained more than a hundred "goose eggs." By my early 40s, I had developed heart disease, hypertension, and prediabetes, which increased the anguish and despondency.

Looking back, I needed proper psychiatric, medical, and spiritual care, but we were too naïve back then to pursue those routes. In fact, not one physician or spiritual mentor during those years of noticeable and significant weight gains ever asked if I might be suffering from an eating disorder. Nevertheless, I am now eternally grateful that I was never drugged by a medical community, or exorcised by a religious community. I was graciously spared both the adverse side effects of some psycho-active meds and potential spiritual abuse.

After desperately praying and seeking a way out of my inner turmoil, my cries for help were heard, and I was graciously deliv-ered. God led me to a path of healing for depression, addiction, and the resulting eating disorder; and it didn't include expensive hospitalizations, a plethora of toxic drugs, or spiritual condem-nation and shame.

I was led to marriage and family therapist Carl Sovine, Ph.D., who skillfully helped me with many of life's issues, including my identity and self-worth—as *God* sees me—and he gave Kurt and me some practical tools to heal and restore our floundering marriage.

Number one, Kurt had to stop the name-calling immedi-ately, which instantly defused the destructive cycle of damaging triggers. Number two, Dr. Sovine worked with him on loving me unconditionally, no matter what size I was at any given time. (And thankfully, Kurt was teachable and has loved me

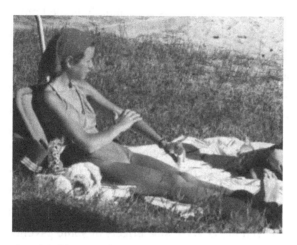

Age 17; 104 pounds (5'8")

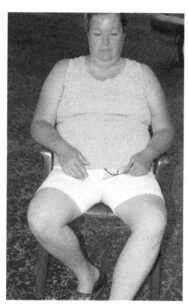

Age 47; 238 pounds (5'8")

unconditionally ever since.) And third, he taught us healthy communication skills that were severely lacking in our relationship.

For example, Kurt and I had developed a terrible habit of yelling at each other when we felt misunderstood by the other person. We were unable to hear what the other had to say. This only escalated the frustrations.

Dr. Sovine taught us to sit on two chairs that were positioned back to back.

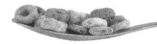

This prevented us from seeing each other's body language. (One can silently scream just by using the right body language!)

Then we had to set a timer for five minutes. We each had a five-minute turn to talk without interruption from the other person. Afterward, we could choose to add additional five-minute time allotments—as long as we each got an equal number of turns to talk. This exercise trained us to really listen to what the other person had to say, without interruption.

We were then able to work on tangible resolutions to disagreements. This simple trick prevented yelling matches that accomplished nothing except to build more walls of miscommunication. Learning to communicate properly put an end to the ongoing tension and strife.

Then I providentially stumbled across Joel Fuhrman, M.D., a board-certified family physician who specializes in nutritional medicine. He is an internationally recognized expert on nutrition and natural healing for eradicating disease, including depression and addiction. In the following chapters, I will explain in further detail how his nutritional information has radically changed my life.

Through both healers, I have found a path to freedom and wholeness.

Now, I consistently eat high-nutrient foods, use proper supplements, exercise, meditate on Scriptures and pray, minimize stress, seek counseling when needed, and make sound sleep a top priority to continue to eliminate depression and addiction.

I have also learned the hard way that when I don't make the healing process a top priority and neglect self-care, or when I indulge in compromises, or allow exceptions, the apathy and carelessness can cause me to relapse into disease and poor health. Most everyone just thinks I'm perpetually on a diet to keep weight off. However, my motivation goes much deeper than a number on a scale.

Due to the rollercoaster ride to hell and back this past decade—which included multiple medical and pharmaceutical errors and the tragic death of a child—I have also experienced enough personal trauma and distress to last a lifetime. Post-traumatic stress can also change the brain and alter its function; therefore, I am gradually healing from that horrific ordeal as well.

I am a firm believer that eating disorders are merely the *symptoms* of underlying conditions, such as malnutrition and food poisoning, depression and addiction, childhood adversity and abuse, learning disabilities, poor body image, low self-esteem, early exposure to dieting, and post-traumatic stress. There is way too much science out there nowadays proving it to believe otherwise.

Proponents of eating in moderation, and critics of abstinence, believe that eating for health is too strict; they feel exceptions can be made for social get-togethers, eating out, special occasions, birthday celebrations, holidays, bereavement—and I get it.

I truly do.

But entanglements and besetments don't work that way. Once addicted to a destructive substance or habit—one bite, one smoke, one injection, one drink, one snort—you can set the chronic disease back in motion. You have to completely abstain from a destructive entanglement.

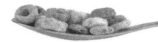

Furthermore, I completely understand the biblical examples of fellowship: "breaking bread together" in both the Old and New Testaments. But back then, food was *not* highly processed and addictive. Modern-day foods are completely abnormal and disease-promoting and contribute to far too many afflictions.

I don't follow Dr. Fuhrman's instructions merely because I want to fit into a pair of skinny jeans for the next class reunion. I follow them because they eradicate *depression and food addiction.* They put an end to myriad other illnesses too: heart disease, hypertension, migraines, diabetes, and cancer, to name just a few. But depression and addiction are the ones that take *me* out.

On holidays and all social occasions out, when others curiously ask, "What are *you* eating?" I graciously answer, "I'm eating foods that heal my body." Period. I know full well that they have absolutely no clue what I am talking about. Nevertheless, that's perfectly fine with me. I follow this path of healing without apology, shame, or others' understanding or approval of it. (During the year I lost a hundred pounds, an acquaintance tried to pry my mouth open to stuff a chocolate éclair into it against my will. Unfortunately, I've experienced similar encounters where others have tried to sabotage my journey to health and wellness.)

I never chose depression and addiction; and I certainly never chose an eating disorder or post-traumatic stress. But each day, I choose healing and freedom from *all of them.*

I refuse to become a victim or wear any affliction as my badge of identity.

On the contrary, I am a victorious overcomer.

I contend daily for optimal health and well-being.

Incredible health, including mental health and performance, is way too precious to me to choose otherwise.

CHAPTER 2

HOW TO ESCAPE FOOD ADDICTION

"Quitting food addiction is uncomfortable,
but so is stopping smoking and quitting cocaine."
Joel Fuhrman, M.D.

It is a good time to be addicted to food. Let me explain.

More than thirty years ago, when I first realized I was addicted to food that was causing me to gain weight and feel miserable, there was scarce information about food addiction. And even if there was, it would have been difficult to access it without the convenience of the internet. Thankfully, due to Dr. Fuhrman tirelessly mining years' worth of scientific studies, he was able to show everyone how to break free from the vicious cycle of it.

Food addiction means biological and chemical dependencies on specific food, mainly sugar, excess fat, and salt.

The only way to stop *any* addiction, including a dependency on food, is to abstain totally, no exceptions. Breaking food addiction requires 100 percent abstinence—there is no other way. Moderation is a myth. Anyone who tells you that eating "just one bite" won't hurt has not studied the science behind food addiction.

According to Dr. Fuhrman, just one bite of an addictive substance activates the dopamine reward system, causing the brain to demand more. Willpower is no match for addictive drives. "The science on food addiction has now established that highly palatable foods, including low-nutrient, high-calorie, intensely sweet, salty, and/or fatty foods which make up the majority of the Standard American Diet produces the exact biochemical effects in the brain that are characteristic of substance abuse."[5]

With all other addictions, such as addiction to alcohol, drugs, or nicotine, there can be a clear line of demarcation never to touch the substance again. But that is not the case with food—we all have to eat.

However, there is a huge and very distinct difference between eating food that our body needs for fuel and eating highly palatable food that is not only addictive, but also disease-causing.

A toxic diet is one that is high in sugar, salt, unhealthy fats, meat, dairy, and processed food. Most Americans are addicted to this way of eating. It is appropriately called the Standard American Diet (SAD), because it consists of the typical food that most Americans eat: eggs and toast, pancakes and sausages, cereal and milk, or granola bars and yogurt for breakfast; a "healthy" sub sandwich, baked chips, and diet soda for lunch; spaghetti, garlic

---

5   Joel Fuhrman, M.D. "'Just One Bite' of Junk Food Fuels
     Food Addiction and Obesity," May 1, 2018, https://
     www.drfuhrman.com/library/eat-to-live-blog/55/
     just-one-bit-of-junk-food-fuels-food-addiction-and-obesity.

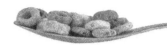

bread, and salad for dinner; and possibly ice cream, yogurt, or cheese and crackers for a bedtime snack.

Dr. Fuhrman says that nearly everyone who has been reared on this typical diet is suffering from food addiction. Food addiction is rampant in our culture. (A small percentage of the population also suffers from eating disorders. I will be discussing eating disorders in a later chapter.) You know that you are addicted to a certain food if you try to "give it up" for New Year's resolutions or when you start a new diet and then a few days later, the cravings are so strong you cave in.

That may have been your experience for years. You know that eating a specific food is detrimental to your health and well-being, but you just can't seem to stop eating it. Kicking a food addiction is much easier than you think if you first understand the science of an undernourished body.

If you have been eating the Standard American Diet for any length of time, your body has become severely malnourished.

Dr. Fuhrman teaches that our bodies were designed to run on micronutrients and chemicals produced by plants. When one is malnourished from a continual diet of low-nutrient food, the nutrient deprivation literally drives overeating.

That is why a typical weight-reduction diet is short-lived. Our bodies were meant to be fueled with superior nutrition—high-nutrient food—not processed meal replacements, "protein bars," and artificially sweetened shakes, sugar-free Jell-O, sugar-free pudding, diet sodas, skim milk, low-fat cottage cheese and yogurt, reduced-calorie pizza, sub sandwiches, chicken breasts, pasta, granola, rice cakes, and reduced fat/reduced sugar ice cream. (Not to mention that artificial sweeteners stimulate the pancreas to produce insulin, which is unfavorable.[6])

He says the buildup of toxins (poisonous metabolites) in the body from lack of micronutrients in the diet creates an addiction that is just as powerful as the addiction to cocaine. And to top it off, he said eating this type of food causes more premature deaths than cocaine![7] Food addiction is a serious matter; don't let the enticing commercials on TV or friends' food porn on Facebook deceive you.

If you are eating low-nutrient food, including an abundance of dairy and animal products, instead of whole, nutrient-rich, plant food—that is a double whammy for disaster because the cravings for fake food will be too overpowering to ignore. You will end up overeating uncontrollably, whether you want to or not. And these excess calories from overeating will fuel disease.

Overeating has little to do with lack of willpower, but a whole lot to do with lack of understanding the healing power of a nutrient-dense diet.

Dr. Fuhrman has created the **A**ggregate **N**utrient **D**ensity **I**ndex, or ANDI food scoring guide. It ranks food according to nutrient density—vitamins, minerals, and phytochemicals. (Phytochemicals are the biologically active compounds found in plants.)[8]

---

6   Joel Fuhrman, M.D., *Eat to Live,* (New York: Little, Brown and Company, Revised edition, 2011), 311.

7   Joel Fuhrman, M.D., "Resolving Food Addiction," Dr. Fuhrman's Health Immersion, October 2012, The Dolce Resort, Basking Ridge, New Jersey.

8   Fuhrman, *Eat to Live*, 64.

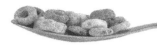

For instance, kale scores 1000, bok choy 865, spinach 707, romaine lettuce 510, broccoli 340, salmon 34, milk 31, whole wheat bread 30, chicken breast 24, pasta 16, corn chips 7, and butter 3.[9] The top "super foods," as he calls them, are green vegetables, beans, onions, mushrooms, berries, nuts, and seeds. They provide our bodies with optimal health and immunity from disease—including food addiction.

To get permanently free from food addiction, he says, we have to flood our body's depleted nutritional stores with high-nutrient food. A goal that he often gives is to shoot for a whole pound of both raw and cooked vegetables; one cup of beans; a serving of cooked, starchy vegetables or whole grains; three to four fresh fruits, including berries; one-fourth avocado (optional); one tablespoon of ground flaxseeds; and one ounce of raw nuts and seeds, such as walnuts, almonds, pine nuts, cashews, sunflower, pumpkin, or sesame seeds every day. (Men may eat two ounces of raw nuts and seeds per day.) Eating all this high-fiber, nutrient-rich plant food will eventually suppress the appetite for unhealthy junk food—and aid in controlling emotional and addictive eating.

At the same time we are flooding our bodies with nutrient-rich food, we also need to completely abstain from eating processed and addictive, low-nutrient food: bagels, bread, chips, crackers, fries, hamburgers, subs, cheese, pizza, sodas, sweets, granola bars, diet food and beverages, grilled chicken, cottage cheese, pasta.

---

9   Joel Fuhrman, M.D., *Nutritarian Handbook and ANDI Food Scoring Guide,* (Gift of Health Publishing, 2012).

When I was trapped in food addiction, I was eating perhaps 200-300 ANDI points per day, at the most. As soon as I began following Dr. Fuhrman's dietary protocol, I was consuming well over 3,000 ANDI points per day!

Is it any wonder I was severely addicted to highly processed food and sweets my entire life? When my body became well-nourished with a variety of nutrient-rich food, the cravings for processed food and sweets subsided. It was as if a switch turned off the runaway motor that was constantly revved up inside me. I was getting the nutrients my body needed for the first time in my life!

Dr. Fuhrman has named this way of eating, the nutritarian diet-style. A nutritarian is someone who eats high-nutrient food in order to meet the body's biological needs for optimal nutrition. Fueling the body with nutrient-dense and plant-rich food eradicates food addiction and numerous other maladies that surface as a result of eating the Standard American Diet.

The one caveat to getting out of food addiction is that the body *will* go through toxic withdrawal for the first several days. It can last for up to three months for some people, depending on how toxic the body has become throughout the years.

This withdrawal phase is critical to understand. Many neglect to comprehend this part—and, sadly, never get out of food addiction as a result.

Most people will feel worse for the first three to four days, not better, but that is a *good* sign. That means the body is getting rid of toxins—and it is not a pleasant feeling. Some of the symptoms of toxic withdrawal, also known as "toxic hunger," may include nausea, vomiting, headaches, growling stomach, bloating, gas,

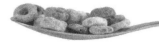

diarrhea, fatigue, weakness, brain fog, sluggishness, anxiety, and irritability. These symptoms are merely toxins being released from storage into circulation for removal, enabling the body to become clean and healthy.[10]

This withdrawal phase can be tough for some people, but it also is relatively short-lived. Additionally, if one does not carefully follow Dr. Fuhrman's nutritional protocol for at least eight to twelve weeks, the taste buds will never adapt and change—and, consequently, will never get to the point of preferring natural, healthy food.

Superior nutrition, eaten consistently for those three months, will radically change your taste buds to the point you will prefer only nutritarian food and no salt. It really does happen if you give it a chance. (This is coming from yours truly, who gagged on greens in the beginning!)

Stick with it, because these months of consistency will also establish meal planning and food prep routines that will become ingrained and automated. The automation will then free your mind to focus on other things.

And, in a relatively short amount of time, you will begin to experience significant improvements in health and energy levels. This newfound energy is highly motivating and will exponentially increase confidence to keep going. This "feel good" attitude propels the passion and desire to maintain excellent health for the rest of your life!

Not giving up during the withdrawal phase is a very small price to pay for getting free from food addiction and enjoying excellent health.

---

10   Fuhrman, *Eat to Live*, 149–159.

If you want to get well, you can. You don't have to live with food addiction and poor health, and you certainly don't have to live life trapped in a body that you no longer recognize. The pleasure one gets from living in this freedom far outweighs anything one may have to give up to achieve it.

It is a privilege to earn one's health back by escaping from food addiction. It is a priceless treasure that money can't buy!

CHAPTER 3

PRACTICAL TIPS
FOR BEGINNERS

"Just do it and don't worry about liking it.
You will love it later!"

Joel Fuhrman, M.D.

WHERE TO BEGIN

I share Dr. Fuhrman's advice, because it has literally transformed my health, my well-being, and my entire outlook on
life—not to mention thousands of other people's lives as well.
And, as I have stated earlier, I did not write this book to create
yet another weight loss memoir that will wind up collecting dust
on a shelf. I have written this book to help anyone permanently
escape food addiction.

Whether one follows Dr. Fuhrman's lectures on PBS or reads
one of his many books, the results will be the same: Individuals
will get rid of food addiction and earn their health back.

The jewel that helped me escape in 2008 was his popular
classic, *Eat to Live.* It is simple, straightforward science that

radically changed my worldview about food. I followed "The Six-Week Plan"—the basic eating plan described in the book.

However, before I started, I spent six weeks studying the entire book. If you just crack the book open to the Six-Week Plan and follow it as any other diet, you may miss the mark, and it may cost you your health in the process.

For instance, five years prior to 2008, I found the Six-Week Plan in *Eat to Live*, but didn't read the rest of the book. I wasn't interested in the science behind toxic hunger, food addiction, optimal health, or longevity. I just wanted a quick way to lose weight and a simple plan to follow.

By the second day, when symptoms of detox started to surface, I caved in and immediately went back to my old way of eating. This continued on and off for the next five years.

When the going gets tough in the beginning—and it will—understanding the science behind cravings, toxic hunger, and withdrawal will enable you to make it through the cravings.

There are no shortcuts.

If you want to become free from food addiction, you must go through the toxic withdrawal phase.

I took a yellow highlighter and studied the entire book as if my very life depended upon it, because it did! (I was sitting on a ticking time bomb of high cholesterol and hypertension.)

And when I came to words such as "sulfur glucosinolates" or "phytochemicals," I jotted them down in a notebook, along with what they did for my body. I kept this running list of words and their meanings so that I could review it from time to time. This was critical information to know, and it helped me achieve

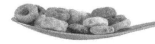

success. As the mind is changed with correct information, the body will transform as a result. Knowledge is power.

(Caution: Because the Nutritarian Diet is so effective in eradicating diseases, such as hypertension and Type 2 diabetes, it is important to be under the care and supervision of a physician if you are taking medications to lower blood pressure and/ or blood sugars.)

THE SIX-WEEK PLAN

The Six-Week Plan in *Eat to Live* will radically change your life *forever!* If you commit to follow it with a steadfast tenacity every day for six weeks—even through possible headaches, brain fog, nausea, or fatigue—you will get rid of the toxins that hold you captive to the addiction.

Your taste buds will also dramatically change. During this time, you will actually begin to taste the subtle flavors in a leaf of romaine lettuce, or the succulent sweetness in a wedge of cantaloupe. When the taste buds change, eating food without salt and sugar becomes a very pleasurable experience.

The cravings for low-nutrient, processed food will significantly dissipate during this time as well. Nearly everyone notices a significant drop in weight afterward, too. I lost twenty pounds in just the first four weeks of following the Six-Week Plan. (I documented my journey with pictures, writings, and medical stats at www.EmilyBoller.com, "Transformation.")

I typed it out using a small font and printed several copies. After trimming excess paper, I had each one laminated at an office supply store. I placed one in my purse, one in my car, one on my desk, one on my bathroom mirror, and one on the refrigerator. I allowed those laminated cards to make all decisions for me, and it worked. A year later, I weighed a hundred pounds less, and no longer suffered from food addiction, coronary artery disease, hypertension, prediabetes, depression, low back pain, cracked heels, and painful boils.

TIPS FOR MAKING IT THROUGH TOXIC WITHDRAWAL

This phase is short-lived; the worst part for many people is the first three to four days. That is the period of time when headaches, growling stomach, nausea, weakness, shakiness, anxiety, irritability, and brain fog are the strongest. Toxic withdrawal may last for up to eight to twelve weeks for some, but the symptoms are significantly reduced.

Dr. Fuhrman calls these symptoms "toxic hunger." Remember, the symptoms are merely toxins being released for removal. This enables the body to become clean and healthy. You *will* feel bad during this time. Expect it so you are not surprised by it. This part takes grit.

If you give in to toxic hunger and eat the food you are craving, the detoxification process will stop—and you will immediately feel better. For instance, if you are experiencing shakiness or weakness and brain fog, and eat a few cookies, or a bowl of cereal and milk, you will soon feel better.

However, you will also regret it, because the sooner you can get to the other side of withdrawal, the sooner toxic hunger will go away. When that happens, you will feel better and start living life to the fullest!

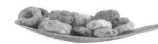
Tips:

- Before you begin, ask your family members for their support by not leaving opened bags of chips or cookies on the counters. Enlist their help in the kitchen so that you are not preparing tempting food. Make your kitchen and home a safe zone.

- Clear your social eating calendar for at least one week. Don't meet up with friends for lunch or dinner during this phase when your cravings will be the strongest.

- Make those laminated cards I suggested earlier and allow them to make all your decisions. Follow this plan, no matter what. A nonnegotiable boundary line is critical to success.

- Choose the highest-scoring, most nutrient-rich food possible to flood your depleted body. Keep a copy of Dr. Fuhrman's *Nutritarian Handbook and ANDI Food Scoring Guide* in your purse, briefcase, or kitchen drawer, and refer to it often. (This helpful tool can be ordered through Amazon.)

- Set a timer for three equally spaced periods of time between your three meals per day. For instance, breakfast at 7 a.m., lunch at noon and dinner at 5 p.m. If you have been in the habit of snacking all throughout the day, this trick will help you "hold out" until the alarm goes off. Once withdrawal is over, you will no longer need to do this, but it is helpful in the beginning to prevent toxic hunger snacking.

✂ When tempted to give in to toxic hunger, call a friend, go on a brisk walk, or simply take a power nap if you are able—do *anything* to distract yourself.

✂ Continually remind yourself that this phase is short-lived and will pass soon.

DITCH THE DIETING MENTALITY

✂ A dieting mentality focuses on all the food one *can't* eat; this deprivation mentality invites self-pity and cheating.

✂ The eating-to-live mentality focuses on all the wonderful food you *can* eat, leading to positivity and enthusiasm!

The Nutritarian Diet is not a crash diet you will go on and off so you can fit into a pair of skinny jeans for a special event. (However, there is certainly nothing wrong with that goal; just don't throw out long-term optimal health and longevity in the midst of the quest.)

Nor is it a weight-loss gimmick that promises you can eat anything you want in moderation and still lose weight. And, thankfully, it is not a restrictive diet in which you count calories or go through meticulous rituals—only to eat everything in sight once the restrictions are lifted.

In fact, just the opposite will occur. Your focus will be on *eating* a plethora of food, full of micronutrients and phytochemicals. When your focus shifts to choosing colorful and life-giving food, you will no longer feel painfully deprived.

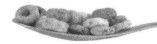

Since I had dieted for most of my life, when I committed to eating this way, it was the first time I felt as though I could actually *eat*—without guilt—instead of *not* eat. When I dieted, my focus was always on what I *couldn't* eat. The deprivation always backfired, and then I would binge eat. Between the malnutrition and the psychological deprivation, I had literally starved myself to obesity.

Instead of my former obsession with counting calories, carbs, and points, I focused on eating plenty of the right kinds of food. For example, according to Dr. Fuhrman, beans are a slowly digested starch—a resistant starch. That means they pass through the small intestine without being digested or absorbed. Because beans digest slowly, they keep you from getting hungry and improve insulin sensitivity. They also make good gut bacteria—a natural probiotic—not to mention they burn fat in the body and bind cholesterol to remove it from the body via the stool. The same goes for raw nuts such as walnuts, almonds, pecans, pistachios, and cashews; they suck saturated fat out of the body as well.

Additionally, he says that the more green vegetables you eat, the more weight you will lose. And when you eat a variety of nuts and seeds (such as sunflower, hemp, pumpkin, sesame, flax, and chia seeds) with greens, it increases the absorption of certain nutrients by *ten* times![11]

---

11   Joel Fuhrman, M.D., *Super Immunity*, (New York: HarperCollins Publishers, 2011), 116.

Understanding this exciting nutritional science is fascinating, and once you comprehend it, it opens up a whole new world of pleasure in eating!

Perhaps for the first time in your life, the focus will get to be on *eating*—instead of *not* eating. Your wilted body will come back to life as you flood it with nutrients.

Also, pitch the "falling off the wagon" mindset. Don't involve any wagons. Wagons are for ponies and children and hayrides—not for getting your health back. That mindset will only set you up for failure, because when you slip up and make a mistake, the brain will automatically think, *I'm off the wagon now, so I might as well throw in the towel for the rest of the day and blow it big-time.*

The wagon mentality can become a trigger for binge eating. You don't want to go there. Instead, at the slightest slip up, recognize and acknowledge it, yet don't make a big deal out of it. Brush it off and immediately keep moving forward. Don't allow a minor lapse in judgment to turn into a major relapse in recovering your health.

WHAT TO DO IF YOU HAVE A FAMILY

I was so addicted, sick, and desperate to get my health back that I didn't care if the rest of my family followed this way of eating or not. I had to put my own oxygen mask on first, so to speak, before I could even think about helping them. Kurt and the kids were supportive of my new adventure, but were totally content with just watching from a safe distance—they had no interest in participating.

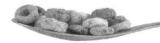

I had a shelf on the refrigerator where I kept my food separate from theirs. It was my safe zone. I did this merely to separate myself psychologically from foods that would no longer serve my goal to get free from the addiction.

By God's grace, I was able to continue to prepare their meat-based entrees. Their meals suddenly had more salads, vegetables, nuts, and fresh fruits added to them—and less bread and fewer sweets—and no one complained, except my then-ten-year-old son. He felt it was unfair that his four older siblings got to eat a lot of junk food when they were his age, and that was a valid complaint from his perspective!

After ten months, and losing nearly a hundred pounds, I gradually quit purchasing processed cereals for my family and replaced cow's milk with almond milk. (Dairy protein boosts the amount of IGF-1 in the blood; IGF-1 stimulates the growth of cancer cells.[12]) I also slowly introduced them to healthier entrees, such as fiesta bean salad and lentil stew—to replace meat entrees—and no one complained. They saw the changes in me and knew the benefits.

Bottom line, don't let having a family be the excuse that you won't be able to get free from food addiction. I am just one of many who have successfully escaped the addiction while having a family who eats the Standard American Diet. It *can* be done!

KEEP THE KITCHEN COUNTERS CLEAN

Yes, you read that correctly.

---

12   Fuhrman, *Eat to Live*, 109.

Before doing anything else, if you haven't already established this habit, I highly recommended starting. Begin by unloading the dishwasher first thing every morning. This simple trick, which takes fewer than five minutes, can make the difference between consistently eating for health and throwing in the towel and quitting. When the dishwasher is empty, there is then a place to put dirty dishes that accumulate throughout the day—freeing up the sink and countertops.

It is much simpler to haul bags of groceries into the house and have a place to put them, or to rinse and cut up vegetables for salad, or to use a blender to make a green smoothie, or to make a pot of soup when the countertops are uncluttered (and the sink is empty of dirty dishes).

In my house, it is also easy for the kitchen counters to become the drop-off place for the daily pile of mail, empty sacks, my purse, gym bags, car keys, the school backpack, and winter coats and hats. I have to work at keeping them clutter-free, but it only takes a minute or two.

Food prep is more inviting and enjoyable when there is a system of organization in the kitchen. If the counters are cluttered with stuff, it is too easy to grab a large handful of nuts, or go to the drive-through, instead of preparing a simple, nutritious meal.

Also, establish the habit of cleaning utensils, knives, blender containers, bowls, and pots as you go. Don't allow dirty dishes to pile up. Wash them as you use them. (Additionally, keep the food in the refrigerator organized as you go too.) A clean, clutter-free, and organized kitchen is a workable kitchen. A little time invested in keeping the kitchen tidy will pay huge dividends of great health.

CHAPTER 4

SET YOURSELF UP FOR SUCCESS

*"It will take strength; it will take effort,
but the pleasures and rewards that you'll get
from a healthy life will be priceless."*

Joel Fuhrman, M.D.

KEEP IT SIMPLE

Four days after I started out on my journey in the summer of 2008, my son with Type I diabetes had a medical crisis that landed him in the hospital. Eventually, he had to be transferred to a children's hospital in a nearby state. I had no idea how I was going to continue to eat healthy without a kitchen, sink, and refrigerator.

But where there is a will, there is always a way.

Just before leaving our home in the middle of the night to make the three-and-a-half-hour drive, I put a cooler in the trunk of the car. I then dumped all the vegetables from our refrigerator's produce drawer into it—and took off.

Every two days, I stocked up on fresh produce and cans of beans at a supermarket close to the hospital. I also purchased a can opener, a paring knife, bags of ice, and one-gallon jugs of water.

The trunk of my car became my kitchen, where I stored and prepped all of my food.

In the hospital parking garage, I found parking spots near drains. I would wash my vegetables over the drains with those gallon-jugs of water.

When it was time for a meal, after preparing it, I put the meal into an empty sack and carried it into the hospital cafeteria.

I ate freshly rinsed leaves of romaine lettuce, green and red peppers, snap peas, cucumbers, tomatoes, carrots, apples, oranges, berries, and almonds. I ate beans straight out of the can.

It worked. I lost forty pounds those first three months—and even more importantly, the cravings for highly salted, sugary, high-fat processed foods had completely vanished by the time I had returned home. Food addiction was gone for the first time in my life!

Whether you have a state-of-the-art kitchen—or just the trunk of your car—you can eat for health, no matter what.

Set yourself up for success by keeping everything simple, especially in the beginning. Don't bite off more than you can chew; otherwise, you may feel overwhelmed and quit. I know men whose wives don't eat this way, and vice versa. They all have found ways to keep it simple and make it work for their individual situations.

The quickest and surest way to change taste buds when first starting out is to stick to vegetables and beans, with the addition

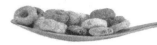

of nuts, seeds, and whole fruits. Even though healthy desserts such as date-sweetened oat bars, date-sweetened brownies, and ice cream made out of frozen bananas and fruit are permissible, they are easy to overeat if you once had a sweet tooth.

It is my personal experience that it is best to stay away from those kinds of desserts, at least in the beginning until toxic hunger symptoms subside. You can always add them later when you are out of the woods, regarding cravings. However, use caution. They may reignite a craving for sweets and overeating.

Cans of drained, unsalted beans, cut-up raw veggies, and fresh berries are convenient to add to salads for quick meals. Bags of defrosted frozen vegetables are great to add to salads as well. I always keep several cans of unsalted beans in the cupboard and bags of frozen veggies and edamame beans (a type of soybean) in the freezer, because they come in handy. I stock up when they go on sale.

A high-speed blender is a wonderful tool for making salad dressings, smoothies, and such, but certainly, it is not a necessity. For the first couple of years, I did fine with an old food processor. I already had the processor, and it was sufficient for making bean dips and smoothies. But when I received a Vitamix for Christmas one year, I could make ice creams and sorbets out of frozen fruits for my family, and creamy dressings and smoothies without chunks of nuts and seeds in them.

Learn to "batch cook" by making a large quantity of food and then putting it into smaller containers. I can make a huge stock pot of vegetable or bean soup in less than two hours on the weekend, from start to finish, and then freeze it into small, individual containers for grab-and-go meals during the week.

Invest in a high-end stock pot with a thick bottom. It is a necessity for making soups, and the pot will last forever.

For protection against hypertension, heart attacks, and strokes, Dr. Fuhrman recommends no more than a thousand milligrams *total* of sodium per day. That means no more than two hundred to four hundred milligrams over and above what is found in natural foods.[13] Therefore, it is important to learn to make vegetable soups and beans without salt.

Here is a simple way to make unsalted beans: Put three cups of dry beans in a large crock pot (any variety of beans will do). Add enough water to cover the beans by at least two inches. Allow the beans to soak overnight. In the morning, add more water to cover the beans generously, and then turn the crock pot on low. By late afternoon, the pot of beans will be fully cooked. Drain any liquid, and voila: a large amount of no-salt beans!

Beans are great for adding to soups, stir fry, and for making dips and hummus. And lentils make a nice replacement for ground beef in chili recipes.

We buy fifty-pound bags of dry beans (and rolled oats) at a local farm store and pour them into five-gallon food storage containers with sealed, airtight lids. I have friends who also purchase nuts and seeds in bulk. Many people order bulk dry goods online.

To prevent getting stuck in a rut, and to open your taste buds to a whole new world of exciting and delicious flavors, it is fun to learn a new recipe every month or so.

Remember, this new eating-style is for the rest of your life, so keep it simple and convenient, at least in the beginning. You

---

13   Fuhrman, *Super Immunity,* 156.

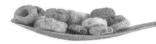

are running a marathon, not a hundred-yard dash. Pace yourself. Stay with it, and don't give up. You will have absolutely no regrets.

As Dr. Fuhrman stated, "It will take strength; it will take effort, but the pleasures and rewards that you'll get from a healthy life will be priceless."

SIX BASIC RECIPES

The following recipes merely serve as a template to help you create your own repertoire of meals. If you want more, Dr. Fuhrman's member center includes thousands of recipes, as well as his *Eat to Live Cookbook*. In addition, simply Google "nutritarian recipes" and you will find a plethora of them.

These recipes are merely guidelines; use any vegetables and salt-free seasonings that *you* prefer or have on hand. The key is to make great-tasting food that you like and will look forward to eating at each meal.

Additionally, the old adage, "Hunger is the best sauce," is true. By omitting snacking, you will increase the pleasure of eating at mealtimes. Once toxic hunger symptoms go away, you will experience true hunger...maybe even for the first time in your life. True hunger really does make eating more enjoyable. And if you have been dieting for most of your life, your world is about to open up to guilt-free *eating,* perhaps for the first time in your life!

If you are inexperienced in the kitchen, please don't let a recipe scare you. It is only a fancy word for different combinations of food. Most of the time, I don't measure ingredients, except for nuts and seeds, but for the sake of consistency, I will provide a general guideline of amounts.

Bottom line, keep it simple. You can keep it uncomplicated *and* healthy at the same time!

BASIC GREEN SMOOTHIE
Serves 2

Ingredients
- A large handful of kale
- A large handful of mixed greens
- 8 ounces water
- 2 tablespoons ground flaxseeds
- ½ ripe avocado
- 2 cups blueberries
- 1 ripe banana

Directions

Grind the flaxseeds first. Then add water and the remaining ingredients. Blend until smooth and creamy.

Tips:

- Green smoothies (aka blended salads) make quick meals on the go. Plus, you can easily flood your cells with a lot of dark, leafy greens this way. If you are rushed at breakfast or lunch, this is a simple and delicious way to consume a nutrient-rich salad on the go.

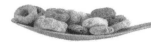

- Feel free to substitute blueberries with almost any fruit and the nuts or seeds with other nuts or seeds that you may have on hand. (Nuts and seeds increase the absorption of greens by ten times. Always eat your greens with nuts or seeds.)

- Greens can be purchased rather inexpensively at the grocery store, or by growing them yourself, even if you just have a tiny yard. Any surplus produce can be stored in plastic bags in the freezer. Frozen greens are great to add to smoothies as well.

- If you don't have a high-speed blender, flaxseeds can also be ground in a coffee grinder.

- When avocados go on sale, stock up on them. Peel and cut them into quarters and freeze them on a cookie sheet. When they are frozen, put them in a plastic bag. This trick is a quick way to add a fourth of an avocado to your smoothie if you have a high-speed blender. Avocados are packed with nutrients and add a creamy texture to smoothies.

BASIC STEAMED VEGETABLES

Ingredients
1 large onion, sliced
1 (12-ounce) box mushrooms
Any vegetable, such as kale leaves, asparagus, broccoli, peppers, or cauliflower

Directions

Fill a 2-quart saucepan with 2-3 inches of water. In the meantime, fill a metal steamer basket or two bamboo steamer baskets with the vegetables. (I use my bamboo steamer baskets almost daily. They can be purchased online.) When the water has come to a boil, place the steamer baskets on top of the pan. Cover. Set timer for 5 minutes. Then turn off the stove burner and allow the vegetables to steam for another 4-5 minutes.

Tips:

- Sometimes I add sliced yams to the mix. Always put the vegetables that take the longest to cook on the bottom.

- Steamed vegetables are delicious served over quinoa.

- When cooked and raw cruciferous vegetables are eaten together at the same meal, it increases their nutritional value.

BASIC BEAN DIP
Serves 8-10

Ingredients

6 cups drained, unsalted cooked beans [or four (15-ounce) cans; any variety]

¾ cup liquid from drained beans

2 tablespoons balsamic or any flavor of vinegar, or fresh lemon juice

3 garlic cloves, chopped

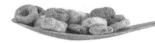

1 tablespoon no-salt seasoning (Southwest chipotle, garlic
& herb, or original blend)

Directions

In a high-speed blender or food processor, add the drained
beans. Add balsamic or apple cider vinegar or lemon juice, and your
favorite no-salt seasoning. Add ¼ cup at a time of liquid from the
beans to create a consistency that you prefer. Blend until smooth
and creamy. Store in an airtight container. Makes 10-12 servings.

Tips:

- As I discussed earlier in the book, all varieties of beans
  are loaded with amazing benefits: They keep you from
  getting hungry, help burn fat, remove cholesterol,
  improve sensitivity to insulin, lower blood sugars, and
  soften stools. Plus, they are inexpensive. Dry beans
  cost about one dollar per pound. One pound of dry
  beans yields about six cups of cooked beans—that's
  less than twenty cents per cup!

- Store-bought hummus or bean dips are expensive and
  usually are loaded with oil and salt. It will sabotage
  weight loss and optimal health. Don't keep it in the
  house. (If you want to make hummus, simply blend
  a can of no-salt, drained chickpeas, a clove or two of
  chopped garlic, the juice of a lemon, and your favorite
  spices until creamy. Many people add tahini paste
  made from sesame seeds, too. The internet has lots of
  hummus recipes; just omit the oil and salt.)

- I like bean dips because I can spread them on cabbage leaves, collard greens, or romaine lettuce leaves—roll them up and wrap a piece of wax paper or foil around them for a quick meal on the go.

- Think outside the box. There are many ways to enjoy bean dips. I even like to mix beans dips into shredded cabbage to make "coleslaw." The sky is the limit when one learns to make a simple bean dip.

BASIC KALE SALAD
Serves 3-4

Ingredients

1 bunch kale leaves, de-stemmed and shredded
1 red pepper, diced
¼ red onion, sliced and diced very thin
1 lemon or lime, juiced (make sure the seeds are omitted)
1 ripe avocado
2 tablespoons raw, hulled sunflower seeds
2 pitted dates (optional)
1 tablespoon no-salt Southwest chipotle seasoning (or any flavor you prefer)

Directions

In a very large mixing bowl, toss together the chopped kale, onions, and red pepper. Set aside. Put the lemon or lime juice, sunflower seeds, avocados, dates, and seasonings into a high-speed blender. Blend until smooth and creamy. With clean hands, thoroughly massage the dressing into the bowl of mixed vegetables. Store leftovers in an airtight container.

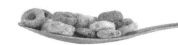

Tips:

- Kale scores 1000 on the ANDI food scoring guide. Kale salad is packed with micronutrients and phytochemicals that prevent plaque from building up in the blood vessels—not to mention that it boosts the immune system and causes the death of cancer cells.

- The salad can be presented beautifully with cherry tomatoes for a garnish.

Basic Vegetable Soup
Serves 12

Ingredients

48 ounces juiced organic carrots (divided in half)

2 (15-ounce) cans diced tomatoes, unsalted

2 onions, diced

4 cloves garlic, minced

4 celery stalks, finely sliced

2 (8-ounce) boxes sliced mushrooms

2 red peppers, diced

4 organic carrots, sliced

2 small zucchinis, sliced

2 bunches kale, thinly sliced (remove stems first)

1 bunch of fresh basil, sliced

1 butternut squash

2 tablespoons no-salt seasoning (original or table blend for starters)

3 (15-ounce) cans no-salt black beans

Directions

Poke several holes on the outside of a clean butternut squash. Microwave the entire squash on high for 16-20 minutes—or until the inside is soft. In the meantime, put ½ of the carrot juice, diced tomatoes, onions, garlic, celery, mushrooms, pepper, carrots, and zucchini in a large stock pot. Bring to a boil and then cover and simmer on low for 25 minutes. After the squash is cooked, scoop out the flesh and put it into a high-speed blender. Add the remaining ½ of the carrot juice and no-salt seasoning. Blend until smooth. Then add the butternut squash mixture to the pot of cooked vegetables, followed by the chopped kale, basil, and black beans. Stir. Simmer an additional 10 minutes.

Tips:

- There is nothing more nourishing, satisfying, and delicious than a bowl of warm soup. In addition, to pack in even more nutrients, I like hot or cold vegetable soups poured over bowls of shredded greens or shredded cabbage. Since greens, mushrooms, and onions are the most powerful against cancer, make sure to include them.

- Soup may seem overwhelming to make at first glance, but it adds a lot of flavor and enjoyment to the nutritarian diet-style. Once you get the hang of it and learn the shortcuts, you will be so glad you persevered and didn't give up.

- Organic carrot juice adds a lot of flavor. It can be purchased in the produce section of most grocery stores.

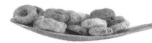

Any vegetable may be omitted or substituted with whatever you may have on hand, but don't skip the organic carrot juice. (Conventional carrot juice is bitter.)

BASIC SALAD DRESSING
Serves 6

Ingredients
- ½ cup raw cashews
- 6 ounces tofu
- 3 cloves garlic, chopped
- 2 celery stalks, chopped
- 2 fresh lemons, juiced (no seeds)
- ½ cup water
- 3 tablespoons nutritional yeast
- Pepper to taste

Directions

Combine all ingredients in a high-speed blender and process until smooth and creamy. Add more water to adjust it to the desired consistency.

Tips:

- Nutritional yeast can be found in most food co-ops or health food stores. It adds a cheesy and savory flavor to foods.

- You can make a plethora of salad dressings from ingredients you may already have on hand. A high-speed blender is able to process the nuts and seeds into a creamy texture. Raw, unsalted cashews or ripe avocados work well for a salad dressing base. Fresh or frozen fruit, citrus fruits, flavored vinegars, and spices add flavor. In a pinch, with a fork, you can even blend tomato paste with balsamic vinegar, almond butter and water.

- Remember from the previous chapter, when plant-based fats are eaten with meals, they increase the absorption of certain nutrients—up to ten times as much! So don't skip nuts and seeds at mealtimes.

- Feel free to improvise with ingredients you may already have on hand. If you have a high-speed blender, you can create a variety of salad dressings. Simply start with a fat source such as nuts, seeds, or avocados. Add an acid such as any flavor of vinegar, lemon juice, orange juice, or tomato sauce. Add a naturally sweet flavor such as a date or two (optional), and flavorings such as spices, herbs, nutritional yeast, celery, and/or garlic—and water for desired consistency.

CHAPTER 5

THE BENEFITS OF SUPPORT

COUNSELING

Life can get overwhelming at times. Occasionally, we get caught in a situation and need help to get through it. Counseling is simply professional guidance in navigating and resolving personal, social, or psychological problems and difficulties.

One of the many benefits of professional counselors is they are bound by law to keep what is shared confidential. This enables the counselee to build a trust with the counselor, and when that trust is established, it enables one to get to the root of issues that are causing havoc in one's life.

Dr. Sovine, who counseled Kurt and me, is a licensed marriage and family therapist. He is highly skilled at listening and then providing tangible recommendations to untangle the messes we present—and his solutions work.

For example, after children came along, Kurt and I struggled with disagreements in front of them, and we knew it was not appropriate or beneficial for them to be listening to our arguments. Dr. Sovine established some clearly defined rules:

1. Absolutely no arguing in front of the children.

2. Never use the bedroom as a place to settle disagreements. (He wanted us to reserve that special room for times of relaxation, refreshment, and intimacy, not marital strife.)

3. Save the laundry list of unresolved issues for him to referee in his office and learn how to find agreeable resolutions.

The tension immediately lifted, and our home became peaceful. With time, Dr. Sovine taught us how to communicate effectively and work through disagreements in a healthy way on our own, without needing his help.

A marriage and home filled with arguments and strife is not conducive to emotional well-being—or to peaceful mealtimes. Being upset is not health-promoting. Although we should never allow our eating decisions to be dictated and controlled by our emotions, if we can significantly reduce emotionally charged triggers, it is extremely helpful.

Even when the biological addiction to food is removed, one can still eat for emotional reasons. These may include numbing psychological and emotional pain, escaping problems instead of finding solutions, escaping responsibilities; and as a sleep aid, to regulate moods, to sedate, or myriads of other reasons that are unrelated to the body's needs for nutrition.

We cannot eliminate all stress and tension from our lives, but we can significantly minimize overcommitments so that we can make time for self-care. A skilled therapist is able to ask the hard questions to pinpoint areas that are out of balance.

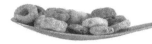

For example, years ago, all five of our children were at home. They were ages eleven, nine, eight, four, and a nursing infant. Between the older children's school, extracurricular activities, sports, recitals, friends, doctor and dental appointments, laundry, and feeding and clothing all of them, I rarely had a free moment to myself.

I was physically drained, spiritually depleted, and emotionally frazzled—and something had to change.

The busyness, chronic sleep deprivation, and lack of time to recharge led to increased emotional eating. I would use food to unwind from the day's stress. After bath times, brushing teeth, and tucking everyone into bed at night, I would seek out the day's leftovers to eat: crusty cheese baked onto the sides of the pan I used to bake lasagna; burnt and chewy roast beef stuck on the bottom of a slow cooker; and bowls of the children's untouched, soggy salads swimming in ranch dressing.

One time, I managed to pull together a birthday party for one of the children and nearly a dozen of her friends (in the midst of nursing the infant). It took every ounce of energy I could muster. That evening, I hit an all-time low and gorged on the leftover pieces of birthday cake and melted ice cream that had been tossed into the trash can.

These unrestrained indulgences became my epicenter of calm. I would get a hit from consuming the high-fat foods, processed carbs and sweets...and then crash on the sofa. My sleep-deprived body was desperately starving for rest, as I continued to starve myself to obesity.

Dr. Sovine opened my eyes to the damage I was doing to myself and helped me devise a practical plan to remedy it. An important part of that plan was enlisting help from Kurt so I could get extra sleep and replenishment on the weekends.

Dr. Sovine also encouraged me to participate in creative sublimation—an activity that would release my pent-up stress in a healthy way. I had developed painting skills years earlier but had suppressed them when children came along. Dr. Sovine said that I had lost myself to my marriage and the demands of rearing a family, which contributed to my out-of-control eating. I resurrected my easel, brushes, and paints and stepped into the creative flow again. He held me to this plan of action until noticeable improvements were achieved. And gradually, I became alive again!

Sometimes, a tangible plan of action from a skilled and trustworthy counselor is necessary to defuse the stresses of life.

Professional counseling is also beneficial for busting lies that create strongholds of deception in one's mind.

I am strongly opposed to animal cruelty and only mention the following story to illustrate a point.

When an elephant is a baby, its trainer ties a heavy chain around its leg. That chain is then tethered to a metal stake in the ground, and when the baby tries to break away, the chain cuts into its skin. The wound causes the babe to hurt worse if it repeats the action by inflicting even more pain. When that happens, the baby elephant finally realizes that it is useless to try to escape, so it quits trying altogether.

By the time the baby elephant grows into an adult, its mind is psychologically tethered to that chain. The elephant can then be tied to a simple hemp rope that is tethered to a wooden stake

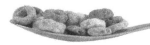

in the ground, and because of the helplessness it had been accustomed to, it will not attempt to escape.

Due to numerous factors, including the verbal abuse I suffered in childhood, I believed a lot of lies about myself. Those lies damaged and severely handicapped my self-image, self-worth, and confidence.

Even experiencing repeated failures became a false belief system for me. If I couldn't do something right, I would throw in the towel and not do it at all. This "all or nothing" perfectionist mentality was not conducive to success at anything, let alone losing weight.

I was like the baby elephant. I had believed many lies, and Dr. Sovine helped me bust free from all of them. A changed mind leads to a transformed life!

EATING DISORDERS

Eating disorders are serious psychological disorders that entail destructive and potentially life-threatening relationships with food. The symptoms may include everything from severely restricting calories (anorexia) to consuming an abnormally large quantity of food in a short period of time—and typically in secret—on a regular basis (binge eating).

After a binge, some may purge the discomfort by self-induced vomiting or very restrictive dieting (bulimia). Others may use laxatives or exercise obsessively in order to prevent weight gain. Many may gain an unhealthy amount of weight in a relatively short period of time—and just keep gaining with each bingeing episode—resulting in obesity-related diseases.

June Hunt, author of *Overeating: Freedom from Food Fixation,* states: "'Bulimia' comes from a Greek word meaning, 'great hunger.' This constant and abnormal appetite of a bulimic is an emotional hunger that no amount of food can fill. They binge in an effort to fill their inner needs and then purge to get rid of the guilt for eating too much, as well as to maintain or lose more weight."[14]

Additionally, overeating blunts the dopamine reward response, encouraging the vicious cycle of more overeating. Dopamine is a neurochemical that regulates motivation and pleasure related to certain stimuli, such as highly palatable foods. Overeating these foods causes a greater desire for them.[15]

In the United States alone, more than twenty million women and ten million men suffer from a significant eating disorder some time in their lives.[16] There are many unreported cases, so that number is actually much higher. It's common to keep eating disorders hidden from others due to the shame and embarrassment of being exposed. I hid my disordered eating for years—even though my fluctuating weight gains and losses were evident.

---

14   June Hunt, *Overeating: Freedom from Food Fixation,* (Torrence, Calif.: Aspire Press, a division of Rose Publishing, Inc., 2014), 17. Used by permission of Rose Publishing, Inc.

15   Joel Fuhrman, M.D. "'Just One Bite' of Junk Food Fuels Food Addiction and Obesity," accessed May 1, 2018, https://www.drfuhrman.com/library/eat-to-live-blog/55/just-one-bit-of-junk-food-fuels-food-addiction-and-obesity.

16   J.L. Hudson, E. Hiripi , H.G. Pope, Jr, and R.C. Kessler. "The Prevalence and Correlates of Eating Disorders in the National Comorbidity Survey Replication," accessed on May 2, 2018, https://www.ncbi.nlm.nih.gov/pubmed/16815322.

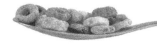

The disorder depends on the way in which an individual is wired. For instance, he or she may be more prone to bouts of depression, anxiety and/or compulsiveness. A part of the disorder is influenced by his or her surroundings, whether the pressure to be thin is extremely important and emphasized a lot. Also, those who suffer with eating disorders are usually experiencing a tremendous amount of unresolved psychological and emotional pain. It takes psychotherapy, along with treating the medical and nutritional needs of the individual, in order to stabilize and recover.

Not only are eating disorders damaging and self-destructive, they lead to a high rate of suicide as well. If you are struggling with an eating disorder, I encourage you to seek professional counseling.

For me, the combination of Dr. Sovine working with me to release years of pent-up emotional pain that I had buried deep within me—followed by adhering to Dr. Fuhrman's nutritional protocol—enabled me to recover from depression, food addiction, and binge eating without taking psychiatric medications.

I had been following the nutritarian diet-style for four years, when suddenly, tragedy struck. My son died. This was at the same time my elderly father was hospitalized in the ICU with pneumonia—and my teenage daughter and I were en route to New York for her to receive a national award at Carnegie Hall.

In the midst of all of this, I was a weight loss success story on *The Dr. Oz Show*. The show was taped in New York City ten days before my son's death and aired two days before his funeral.

I suddenly felt as if I had been tossed into a washing machine on spin cycle, on top of experiencing the profound and excruciating anguish of losing a child.

I had no idea what was about to hit me in the days and months to come. The impact of a child's death is like none other; it is appropriately called "complicated bereavement" for a reason. Plus, as my son's primary caregiver, I had just spent five very stressful years walking the tightrope of never-ending trauma as a result of multiple medical and pharmaceutical errors made in his case. During one such episode, he attempted to gouge one of his eyes out to put an end to hallucinations that he had been experiencing and got his entire index finger stuck inside the eye socket.

After the initial shock of his death wore off and the funeral was over, my world turned completely dark in a vale of tears. I lost my appetite. I was exhausted, yet I couldn't sleep. I had nightmares. My legs felt as if they were filled with bags of sand from the weight of grief, and I could barely get out of bed, let alone brush my teeth. I lost all desire to carry on.

When I was in public, I would randomly cry in front of complete strangers...including in the middle of the produce section at the grocery store. It was embarrassing and exhausting to be in public, so I hibernated in the safety of my home. The intensity of the trauma was so overwhelming that I temporarily lost control of my bowels. I was a mess physically, mentally, and emotionally.

As a result, I could not muster the wherewithal to buy and prepare food or eat correctly. The post-trauma stress and depression were suffocating the life out of me. I didn't revert back to eating the Standard American Diet, but I did neglect eating dark, leafy greens and beans as my main source of nourishment.

Instead, I ate bowls of oatmeal with peanut butter—high-calorie, low-nutrient sources of energy. I preferred oat bars

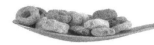

sweetened with dates that were stored in our freezer, and chocolate ice cream made from frozen bananas and cocoa powder.

This cumulative stress on my body, physically, mentally, and emotionally, ignited the depression and binge eating disorder all over again. Apathy set in, as I became emotionally detached—a coping mechanism for self-preservation. I started mindlessly bingeing on low-nutrient plant foods such as nuts, oat bars, frozen banana ice creams, store-bought hummus made with salt and oil, whole wheat tortillas with peanut butter spread on top, and bowls of unsalted popcorn. I was trapped in the addiction once again.

My new clothes didn't fit anymore. The increasing numbers on the scales added an extra layer of grief to my already-shattered heart. The weight loss success story began to unravel right before my and everyone else's eyes. Additionally, with each pound gained, my anxiety level skyrocketed...along with a suffocating phobia of being seen in public.

Others were gracious and understanding, but I felt ashamed of my lack of fortitude and self-control—not realizing at the time that I was running away from processing the trauma and grief. Finally, I hit a wall and couldn't go on.

I had lost my footing and struggled to get back on the path of freedom. But, thankfully, I had enough self-awareness and knowledge to know that path back to recovery and healing. It wasn't an instant turnaround. I struggled immensely at times under the heaviness of complicated bereavement, but I slowly put one foot in front of the other.

Dr. Sovine recommended that I quit weighing myself, at least for a season, so the higher numbers on the scales wouldn't trigger anxiety-ridden bingeing episodes. I stayed the course of eating greens, beans, nuts, seeds, and berries again.

With time, the depression lifted and the binge eating gradually subsided. But right when I was making consistent progress toward recovery and feeling better, my mother passed away. Then, another traumatic event happened in my personal life that was beyond my ability to cope—which landed me on the phone with a suicide prevention hotline counselor. And then about a year later, my father died.

This time, I was more proactive in reaching out for help as quickly as possible. I scheduled additional appointments with Dr. Sovine; plus, I added grief counseling at a local community center. In addition, Kurt and I started attending a small group ministry through our church in order to heal internally from the layers of pain. All of this helped me process and navigate the tsunami of emotions that were overtaking me. I even added massage therapy to the recovery toolbox.

I continued to follow Dr. Fuhrman's nutritional and lifestyle protocols for treating depression and food addiction; this included not only the nutrient-rich diet, but also morning light therapy—an effective treatment in which an individual uses a special fluorescent light or morning sunshine in order to prevent or treat depression—sound sleep every night, exercise, and proper supplementation. I clung to the treatment plan with fervency.

Now, I am eating only nutrient-rich vegetables, beans, berries, nuts, and seeds, and I'm recovering again. I learned the hard way that I cannot stray from the path of healing by making exceptions, including trauma or bereavement. The pounds I had

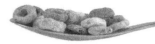

regained are coming off, the paralyzing weight of complicated bereavement is lifting, and I am now genuinely happy to be alive again.

I share all of this to encourage anyone who is currently suffering from trauma, profound loss of any kind, or an eating disorder—or knows someone who is suffering—there is hope. With proper care, broken and traumatized hearts can heal. Eating disorders can dissipate. Recovery is possible.

A note of caution: Eating disorders really are life-threatening illnesses that require professional help for recovery. However, some eating disorder treatment professionals have unofficially labeled *healthy eating* "orthorexia."

While it may be true that some could push even healthy eating to an obsessive extreme, the majority of people never go to such extremes unless they have deeply ingrained and unre-solved psychological issues to overcome—which has nothing to do with food per se. The unofficial orthorexia label can do more harm than good if one doesn't understand the science behind food addiction and what makes up good health.

Dr. Fuhrman has addressed this topic in "Ask the Doctor" on his member center site, because orthorexia has circulated in the news and on Facebook at various times throughout the years. He said there is no such thing as orthorexia, because a person who is truly into *healthy eating* would not restrict his or her calorie intake to become too thin and malnourished—that is an oxymoron of what healthy eating is all about! Optimal health involves maintaining a favorable muscle and skeletal mass, too.

The idea that omitting "normal food" (i.e.: junk food/fast food) from one's diet is pathologic—and that promoting a healthy emotional outlook on food should include eating whatever one desires—is misguided and irresponsible.

Dr. Fuhrman has said many times that encouraging people to eat disease-causing foods, just because it is socially acceptable, is no better than promoting smoking as a socially acceptable pastime or giving people a negative diagnostic label who do not smoke or use drugs or alcohol.

Those who support spontaneous and intuitive eating actually support having sweets and hamburgers if one desires them. They confuse "normal eating"—eating the same foods that most Americans eat—with foods that promote health and well-being, including optimal mental health. "Unhealthy foods alter our brains in ways that make us emotionally attached to the very foods that are doing us the most harm."[17]

In addition, it is a scientifically proven fact that eating highly palatable foods—sweet, salty, fatty food such as the Standard American Diet—will trigger the vicious cycle of overeating. "Our level of susceptibility to addictive behaviors varies by genetic predisposition and emotional state. Nevertheless, highly palatable food has physiologically addictive properties that will make almost anyone experience a lack of control."[18] Eating these "normal" foods causes a greater desire for them. And, as I wrote earlier, eating highly palatable foods and animal products

---

17   Joel Fuhrman, M.D., *Fast Food Genocide*, (New York: HarperCollinsPublishers; 2017), 11.

18   Fuhrman, "'Just One Bite' of Junk Food Fuels Food Addiction and Obesity," May 1, 2018, https://www.drfuhrman.com/library/eat-to-live-blog/55/just-one-bite-of-junk-food-fuels-food-addiction-and-obesity.

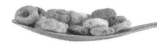

contributes to developing diabetes, heart disease, depression, autoimmune diseases, hypertension, cancer, and myriad other diseases. There is absolutely nothing normal about having one's chest cut open to bypass clogged arteries or having a limb amputated due to diabetes complications.[19]

All of this misguided information illustrates just how pervasive and ingrained self-destructive food habits are in our culture—even in some recovery programs. One must pay attention to the dietary quality of food or cravings will be too intense to ignore.

Food addiction is a serious issue and eating disorders are progressive illnesses—meaning they get worse over time—so the quicker they are halted, the quicker the damage to all the organs is stopped and repair and healing can begin.

SUPPORT GROUPS

Back in 2008, as soon as I decided to commit to the nutritarian diet-style with both feet in, I knew that making major changes happens best in communities of support. I also knew that I would need outside help to overcome the powerful food addiction. And it wasn't just the biological addiction to the Standard American Diet—I had to overcome the social pressure to eat it as well.

I live in the Midwest, where it is expected to eat meat and potatoes, pancakes and sausages, pizza and chicken wings. In fact, my hometown of Fort Wayne, Indiana was ranked the most

---

19   Fuhrman, *Fast Food Genocide*, 1-8.

obese city in the nation in 2017![20] We even have a festival every summer where an entire section of the downtown is reserved for food trucks. It is aptly called "Junk Food Alley."

However, my mind was made up. Nothing was going to deter me. I joined Dr. Fuhrman's member center and had immediate access to hundreds of like-minded people who cheered me on to victory.

I was able to ask questions and receive answers from those who had successfully overcome food addiction and earned health back. I asked questions such as, "I'm hosting a birthday party this weekend. What tips does anyone have to offer?" or "Help! I'm having a craving for chocolate, what should I do?" The synergy of support was invaluable.

I also had direct access to Dr. Fuhrman via "Ask the Doctor," a place where members are able to send questions to him or one of his associates and receive an answer within a day or two, when I had medical questions. And I had plenty of them, especially that first year.

He helped me navigate toxic withdrawal symptoms.

He reassured me after I experienced some minor hair loss (due to hormonal changes) that it would only be temporary and that my hair would grow back even thicker. And sure enough, it did.

He coached me through a major surgery—a hysterectomy. He taught me how to continue to eat throughout the recovery process afterward so that I would continue to lose weight.

---

20   Jonathan Shelley. "Study rates Fort Wayne 'fattest city in America.'" WPTA21, accessed September 12, 2018. http://www.wpta21.com/story/36188308/study-rates-fort-wayne-fattest-city-in-america.

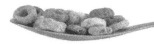

And he guided me through the rollercoaster ride of careless medical and pharmaceutical errors that happened to my son, who had Type I diabetes.

The member center support has been invaluable to my success in not only getting out of food addiction, but also in staying free. And after my son died, it was the members' outpouring of support, and Dr. Fuhrman's expert advice, that helped me through the ups and downs of the post-trauma and bereavement. Their ongoing support was literally lifesaving at times.

Now, there are several "Eat to Live" support groups on Face-book. Social media has been a wonderful tool for many to get the community of support they need.

Many, including myself, have organized local nutritarian support groups. I have facilitated several at libraries. Others have led them at their local Y or in their churches and homes.

I have friends in Florida who have shared a potluck meal together, consisting of their favorite nutritarian recipes, once a month for the past six years. They rotate it, so everyone shares a turn at hosting it, and they also take turns preparing a brief presentation for each gathering.

At their last gathering, someone demonstrated how to make nutritarian cheese. Other times they have discussed a topic from a book or video or have had a guest speaker.

All it takes is a couple of people who want to get together and support one another. Don't wait until the day you find a support group—start one!

I have absolutely no regrets about reaching out for support since the day I began this journey. I am free from food addiction today *because* of the ongoing and consistent support I have received from many throughout this entire time.

SPIRITUAL CARE

After the whacko experience with those women praying for me years ago, I eventually found a healthier group of like-minded friends. They supported me with their prayers and encouragement.

If anyone reading this has been spiritually wounded by those who claim to be messengers of the Most High, I am truly sorry, because that is not His heart. In fact, the Lord is described as a Good Shepherd in Psalm 23 who tenderly cares for his sheep. And He is all about seeing us become victorious over *any* entanglement—because He sees our potential and wants us to become the *best* that we can be! He is our biggest fan and cheerleader!

Just this past week, someone sent the following to me: "I have all the books in the world, but I cannot seem to discipline myself to do what I have to do." This is a commonality among a lot of people with whom I have interacted.

My faith is the foundation of my life. Faith has brought me through some excruciating pain at times, and I can honestly say that one of God's specialties is that *He rescues*.

"The righteous person may have many troubles, but the LORD delivers him from them all."[21] "The LORD is close to the brokenhearted and saves those who are crushed in spirit."[22]

---

21   Psalms 34:19, King James Version.
22   Psalms 34:18, New International Version.

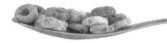

"He raises the poor from the dust and lifts the needy from the ash heap."[23]

One of the most afflicted persons who ever walked on the face of this Earth was a man named Job. He was a wealthy man with a large family (ten kids!), many employees, and extensive flocks. Then one day four messengers came to tell him very tragic news. He had lost everything—*everything*—except his wife. (I can't begin to fathom the complicated bereavement that ensued.)

If that wasn't enough trauma and loss, he then suffered terrible boils from head to toe. Job's life was bleak and miserable as he cried out, "My eyes will never see happiness again...I despise my life...my days have no meaning."[24]

His wife wanted him to curse his Maker and die (after all, she had lost all of her dear children and wealth, too), but Job refused. His so-called friends then spouted some utterly stupid and ridiculous comments, which only added to his confusion and pain.

Finally, Job resolved to continue to honor God and avoid evil, in spite of all the anguish and suffering. Eventually, Job was healed, and everything was restored to him; including the same number of children and even more wealth than before. He said, "Those who suffer he delivers in their suffering; he speaks to them in their affliction."[25]

Life is hard. It is full of troubles at times, but the Lord's specialty is help and rescue. Even addiction is not too difficult

---

23   I Samuel 2:8, NIV.

24   Job 7:6-16, NIV.

25   Job 36:15, NIV.

for Him. I have learned that His teachings contain gold nuggets for getting out, and staying out, of addictive entanglements.

As I shared previously, my childhood created the perfect petri dish for food addiction to develop. I didn't choose to have a food addiction by the age of six—any more than I chose to have blue eyes instead of brown. But thankfully I was led to a path of deliverance and healing. It is now *my choice* to walk out of it or not.

God's plans are to help us prosper and not to harm us; to give hope and a future.[26] His plan is *not* for us to suffer in our addictions and diseases.

We all have this little part of us called an ego. There are different names for it: the flesh, old man, carnal nature, sinful nature, evil desire, sin, earthly nature, old self. Some even call it the addictive monster or squealing pig within.

Basically, it is the lustful wants and desires within us that oppose the wonderful creation that we were originally designed to be. This sinful nature is wired for indulgence—and gains strength that way—and makes war against the very purposes of life itself.

For simplicity's sake, I'll just call this destructive little monster "the flesh."

The flesh—it does not willingly submit; in fact, it *cannot* submit. It does its own thing.

Deep down, we want to do what is right, we really do, but inevitably, we stray and mess up. We have the desire, but we cannot seem to carry it out. It is as if there's another force within

---

26   Jeremiah 29:11, paraphrased.

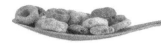

us at war with our minds. This epic conflict is why we end up struggling as we do.[27]

So how do we escape this hopeless captivity?

God's Spirit empowers us to have victory over the flesh.

In other words, the mighty strength of His Spirit can enable us to overcome the pull of the flesh—no matter how strong the addiction. And when we meditate on Scriptures and pray, and then by faith obey what we are shown, that act of humility and obedience begets even more power and control over the flesh.

When we continually deny the flesh what it wants, we grow spiritually stronger and those ugly, lustful desires weaken and then eventually die out.

And this strong spirit sustains us when we encounter life's troubles.[28]

All of the above includes wisdom and common sense. When we apply this practical sensibility, success follows, and we are spared a lot of unnecessary angst. The following biblical quotes are some of my favorites, simply because they have proved helpful in keeping me out of food addiction:

- "Do not think about how to gratify the desires of the flesh."[29]
  - In other words, it's not wise for anyone escaping food addiction to hang out at the doughnut shop, linger in the candy aisle, visit the kitchen late at

---

27 Romans 7:14-25, paraphrased.
28 Proverbs 18:14, paraphrased.
29 Romans 13:14, English Standard Version.

night, or keep ice cream and chips in the house. For me, I have found that brushing and flossing my teeth after the evening meal—and then staying out of the kitchen for the rest of the night—minimizes temptations to gratify the flesh. I also don't keep ice cream in the house. I'm not going to give the flesh an opportunity for gratification; even though cravings for it subsided years ago.

- "Do not join those who drink too much wine or gorge themselves on meat, for drunkards and gluttons become poor, and drowsiness clothes them in rags."[30]
  - The old adage "show me your friends and I'll show you your future" is true. We really do need to be mindfully aware of who we hang out with on a regular basis. Self-destructive drinking and eating not only ruins our health but affects our alertness, energy levels, productivity, financial resources, and self-esteem. As with all self-destructive addictions, it may become necessary to cultivate new friends if current ones are leading us down a dangerous road.

- "Mark out a straight path for your feet; stay on the safe path."[31]
  - In order to live in freedom, it's important to establish clearly defined boundary lines that produce

---

30   Proverbs 23:20-21, NIV.
31   Proverbs 4:26, New Living Translation.

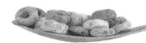

predictable and consistent results...and then stay within those lines, no exceptions. Simply put, we must have a plan and then stick to it, no matter what. There is safety and freedom within boundaries.

- "You need guidance to wage war, and victory is won through many advisers."[32]
  - Reaching out to others for guidance helps us become victorious over food addiction. We just need to make sure that advice lines up with science instead of opinions and pop culture.

- "Let your eyes look straight ahead; fix your gaze directly before you."[33]
  - We can't let anything or anyone sidetrack us from our goals. We must keep our eyes on the prize.
  - You are not facing any temptation that others haven't already faced. But there is always a way out to get through it without succumbing to it.[34]
  - With every temptation, there is always a way out. If we look for the escape hatch, it's there for us to escape!

- "Do not be wise in your own eyes; fear the LORD and shun evil. This will bring health to your body and nourishment to your bones."[35]

---

32   Proverbs 24:6, NIV.
33   Proverbs 4:25, NIV.
34   I Corinthians 10:13, paraphrased.
35   Proverbs 3:7-8, NIV.

EMILY BOLLER

- "Sin is crouching at your door; it desires to have you, but you must rule over it."[36]
  - We must ignore the doorbell if "the flesh" rings!

- "'I have the right to do anything,' you say—but not everything is beneficial. 'I have the right to do anything'—but I will not be mastered by anything."[37]
  - We can eat *anything* we desire, but not everything is beneficial for us. Science has now proven both the destructive and addictive properties of disease-causing food.

- "When you sit to dine with a ruler, note well what is before you, and put a knife to your throat if you are given to gluttony. Do not crave his delicacies, for that food is deceptive."[38]
  - Deceptive food is misleading: Grandma's award-winning chocolate fudge brownies, deviled eggs, and sugar cream pie. That kind of food will entangle and create diseases that will eventually suck the life out of us. We must kill cravings before cravings kill us!

- "Fear of man will prove to be a snare."[39]
  - I've learned through mistakes that I cannot allow the fear of what others may think or say dictate

36 Genesis 4:7, NIV.
37 I Corinthians 6:12, NIV.
38 Proverbs 23:1-3, NIV.
39 Proverbs 29:25, NIV.

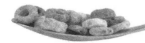

what I put into my mouth. I cannot make compromises in order to please others.

- "Forget the former things; do not dwell on the past."[40]
  - ○ If an impulsive slip up or lapse in judgment happens—and I've had hundreds of them, even throughout the year I lost a hundred pounds—brush it off, move on immediately, and do not dwell on the mistake. That is what Olympic champions do. [41]

- "Even youths grow tired and weary, and young men stumble and fall; but those who hope in the LORD will renew their strength. They will soar on wings like eagles; they will run and not grow weary, they will walk and not be faint."[42]
  - ○ As we keep putting one foot in front of the other, the LORD will keep renewing our strength and amazing results will eventually happen. Freedom from food addiction is possible for *everyone!*

Let's all soar like the eagles!

---

40   Isaiah 43:18, NIV.
41   Lanny R. Bassham, *With Winning in Mind: The Mental Management System,* (BookPartners, Inc., 1995).
42   Isaiah 40:30-31, NIV.

CHAPTER 6

INSPIRATIONAL WRITINGS

HOW AN INTERNET TROLL CHANGED MY LIFE

Back in the summer of 2008, when I started my journey to get my health back, I never intended to be an inspirational blogger or speaker. In fact, I didn't even know what a blog was.

I had been busy rearing five children for nearly two decades and didn't have a portable device or laptop. I had a PC and knew how to use Word and connect to the internet—and that was about it. I didn't even know how to cut and paste.

I had joined Dr. Fuhrman's member center that year because I knew that I would need the support. I started a documentary journal and called it "Journey of Transformation."

It was a place for me to record my journey, including my victories and struggles, and others could view it as well. The members were just as happy as I was when I escaped a temptation or lost another pound. My weight loss was a team effort of victories!

By the following summer, I had lost a hundred pounds, and Dr. Fuhrman asked if I would write a short essay about my

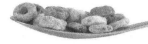

favorite vegetable for his (now former) blog, "Disease Proof." I submitted the piece and his audience of readers enjoyed it.

Then he asked if I could submit some previous writings from my journal on the member center. After tweaking the works a bit, I submitted those as well, and once again, his readers enjoyed them.

It was fun, but I didn't consider myself to be a blogger—until an internet troll entered the picture.

The troll was disguised as four males and five females and began posting mean and nasty comments about my posts. This continued for three months, and I almost quit blogging several times. I think readers started following my posts just to view the nasty comments! All nine identities were traced to the same internet address. Eventually, the troll was exposed, and the derogatory comments immediately stopped.

What started out as a simple piece about my favorite vegetable snowballed into writing a weekly post on Dr. Fuhrman's blog for more than *four years!*

Throughout that time, I also met and interviewed some incredible people from all over the nation who had also earned their health back. I posted those interviews on the blog as well.

For example:

- A middle-aged woman had suffered from incapacitating psoriasis for more than thirty years. She also suffered terrible side effects from the toxic medications she was taking to alleviate it. Today, she has beautifully clear skin without any medications.

- A woman was bedridden, taking nearly thirty medications, and unable to function by her late twenties as a result of lupus. After she changed her diet, her blood tests became normal, and she was able to get off all medications, except one. She is now working in a fulfilling career.

- A middle-aged man had quadruple bypass surgery and a stent procedure two years later to unblock clogged arteries. Afterward, he woke up in the recovery room with shortness of breath and was sent home to get his affairs in order—and prescriptions for over six hundred dollars' worth of medications per month (out-of-pocket expenses). He lost 140 pounds within one year, no longer needed medications, and became the epitome of health and fitness.

- A middle-aged woman had ovarian cancer and was told by two physicians that she only had a few months to live. Instead, she decided not to accept that fate and over-came the cancer by flooding her body with high-nutrient foods—and that was more than nineteen years ago!

- A young father lost 333 pounds and was no longer house-bound. He became an avid cyclist and rode his bike year-round.

- A middle-aged man was taking four medications for asthma and used an inhaler every morning. By following the nutritarian protocol, he no longer had asthma and was free of all medications.

- A young mother had been suffering the physical and emotional pain of cystic acne and had been seeing dermatologists and taking meds for it since age sixteen.

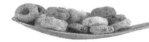

Because of her diet change to nutrient-rich foods, she was finally able to enjoy clear skin again.

The list above is just a sampling of people I had interviewed. Many of them, I had the privilege of meeting in person. I was blown away by their testimonies. I had witnessed firsthand how food had the power to restore damaged bodies to health and wholeness.

During those four years, I also traveled and gave inspirational talks. Some of the gigs were at Dr. Fuhrman's health getaways and weekend immersions, and others were on television and in churches. At one of the getaways he introduced himself as having the book smarts and me as having the street smarts. (My education has been from the School of Hard Knocks!)

One event in particular that I looked forward to was a company's biannual health retreat. The employees would arrive on Sunday afternoon from all over the country and then fly back to their various destinations the following Saturday.

Throughout the week, they were fed delicious, nutritarian meals as they simultaneously experienced detoxification from the Standard American Diet. I would emcee the event, and from my vantage point at the front of the lecture room, I could see their countenances change as the week progressed.

On Mondays and Tuesdays, their faces would be downcast and the room's atmosphere would be filled with a lethargic fog. I could tell they were suffering from the ill effects of toxic hunger and withdrawal.

On Wednesday afternoons, they hiked at a nearby state park to help get them through detoxification. By Thursday mornings, almost everyone would enter the lecture room happy and laughing, and their faces would be lit up!

We always enjoyed line dancing on Thursday evenings, and by that time, the same room would be filled with enthusiasm and joy! When they left on Saturday mornings, almost everyone had lost a significant amount of weight.

Many of them, who had previously been taking blood-pressure-lowering drugs or oral diabetic meds, no longer needed them. (They were carefully monitored and supervised by Dr. Fuhrman and his associate, Dr. Jay Benson, the entire week.)

After years of meeting so many people from all walks of life, listening to their stories, and watching them transform before my very eyes, I am changed.

- I met a couple whose children practically had to rear themselves, because the parents were too overweight, sick, and incapacitated to care for them properly.

- I listened to a young mother who could no longer muster the strength to perform daily responsibilities due to food addiction.

- I met several individuals who were suicidal due to the hopeless entanglement of food addiction.

- I met a man who could no longer climb a ladder to fix his home's maintenance problems due to obesity.

- I met a young woman who had to drop out of college due to a soda addiction.

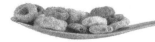

As a result of all these experiences, I will never be the same again. Food really does have the power to destroy a life—or to heal and restore a life.

"Disease Proof" (Dr. Fuhrman's former blog) is no longer online, so my posts cannot be accessed anymore. However, I have selected a few of them to include in this chapter.

Dr. Fuhrman wrote the following about my blog posts in his book *The End of Dieting* (2014) where several of them were published: "You are not alone in your struggle with your weight and food addictions. A successful nutritarian and contributor to my blog since 2009, Emily has inspired thousands of people to change their lives."[43]

May you be challenged and inspired by them too.

IT TAKES COMMITMENT

Success has nothing to do with economic status, nationality, education, social standing, professional training, career choice, a stable upbringing, or even support from love ones. Success is a direct result of thoroughly studying, understanding, and assimilating the science behind Dr. Fuhrman's nutritional recommendations—and then making the decision to earn your health back, no matter what.

Success is having both feet in the nutritarian diet-style at all times, not straddling the fence by eating high-nutrient foods during the week and indulging on the weekend or eating for

---

43   Joel Fuhrman, M.D., *The End of Dieting*, (New York: HarperCollins Publishers; 2014), 92.

health only when it is convenient. All who have succeeded made the firm decision to commit fully.

WHAT IS YOUR JACK DANIEL'S?

I make it my mission to read *Drunkard*, by Neil Steinberg, every couple of years. The book was the impetus for my transformation, because it demolished my concrete wall of denial. It forced me to face the ugliness of my food addiction head-on.

Every time I now read it, something new pops out. One time, it was Steinberg's description of his moment to unwind after work, at the bar, just before drinking his favorite glass of Jack Daniel's. I could totally relate to it.

Years ago, when I was obese, my "Jack Daniel's" was the leftovers after the evening meal. I loved to unwind from the day and soothe my frazzled nerves by mindlessly eating, even though my stomach was full. The twirling universe stopped at those moments for me; it was my calm epicenter in the midst of my too-busy life.

If I'm not careful, Jack can still creep into my life—if I am not keenly aware of his tactics. He is hiding in the dark crevices; but as long as I continue to shine the flashlight on him, and continue to expose him, he can't and won't harm me!

Exposing Jack makes him powerless, because he is a coward in the light. Don't give him the pleasure of lulling you into believing that he is your epicenter of calm. That is a lie.

What is *your* Jack Daniel's? Do you use food to regulate emotions...to calm your nerves, de-stress, sedate, or soothe pain?

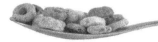

If so, it's time to walk out of the darkness and into the light; it's time to be set free!

PERSPECTIVE DETERMINES OUTCOME

Those who succeed with the nutritarian protocol view it as an *opportunity* to "earn" health back. Their perspective is different from those who focus on all the foods they may be giving up for the rest of their lives.

Instead, those who succeed focus on giving up diabetes and injections of insulin, heart disease and open-heart surgery, toxic and expensive medications, and scheduling life around medical appointments. This different perspective enables them to get past toxic cravings in order to enjoy great tasting foods, in their natural state.

Conversely, those who repeatedly fail have the mindset of dieting. They view the nutritarian approach as just another diet designed only to lose weight—and, subsequently, their focus is on restriction and deprivation. This mentality invites self-pity and cheating. And repetitive cheating doesn't allow taste buds to change or to break free from the vicious cycle of toxic hunger.

CHANGE A MISTAKEN IDENTITY

People become what they believe to be true about themselves and what they repeatedly tell others. If individuals believe they are failures, they will fail. If they tell everyone that they are a compulsive overeater, they will compulsively overeat in times of stress.

It is vitally important to declare and believe in an identity congruent with what you want to be. If you want to be someone who eats healthy food, then don't be afraid to tell others. Don't be ashamed to eat a salad when everyone else at the table is eating lasagna. You don't have to be rude or obnoxious about it—but when asked, don't be afraid to say that you enjoy eating food that makes you feel well. What you believe about yourself is what you will become.

AVOID THE MODERATION MYTH

When it comes to toxic food, there is no such thing as eating in moderation. For someone struggling with a food entanglement, taking one bite of an addictive food can be just as dangerous as smoking one cigarette for a former nicotine addict. Don't believe the moderation myth that you might hear from physicians, counselors, ministers, friends, co-workers, or relatives.

The truth is that just one bite of an addictive food can do great harm. It is much easier to keep addictive cravings extinguished than to be continually fighting obsessive compulsions. It only takes a tiny spark to reignite a food addiction, so eradicate moderation from your vocabulary.

THERE ARE NO SHORTCUTS

Everyone has to cross the threshold of withdrawal from toxic foods, which, for most people, is no fun. Toxic hunger can be unpleasant. You might experience headaches, nausea, weakness, fatigue, shakiness, and irritability that can last several days.

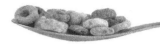

But once the symptoms have been resolved, and if you no longer consume toxic foods, the symptoms don't return.

Also, salt is a particularly tough habit to kick for some, but once the addiction to salt is gone, taste buds change, and the subtle flavors of fruits and vegetables in their natural state become highly enjoyable.

TOMORROW NEVER COMES

Waiting until after the holidays or a special occasion to begin eating for health is a misleading idea. Telling yourself you will "start tomorrow" is a lie. There is always another celebration or family event.

After Thanksgiving, Hanukkah, and Christmas comes the Super Bowl, followed by Valentine's Day, Passover, Easter, Mother's Day, graduation parties, multiple birthday parties, a wedding or two, a Father's Day cookout, summer barbecues and picnics, vacations, county fairs, fall festivals, Halloween, and then the year-end holidays all over again.

You must make the firm decision to eat for health each day and hold fast to that commitment, no matter what the calendar says.

THE REFRIGERATOR IS NEVER THE SOLUTION

Eating is never a solution to any problem. Emotional health is never achieved via the refrigerator, cupboard, or drive-through window. Life is full of ups and downs, joys and sorrows, pleasures and pains; that is why our lives are interesting and, ultimately, fulfilling. Address emotional issues by talking to a professional counselor, a trusted family member or friend, or join a support group. Addictive food and drugs are never the solution.

ABSTINENCE IS IMPORTANT

Abstinence is staying within a clearly defined boundary line. The purpose of an established boundary line is to keep one safe. In that safe place is freedom from addiction and disease.

Food addiction can be as serious as alcoholism and drug addiction. It destroys lives. A commitment to abstain from all processed food and junk food is necessary. Abstinence is radical, but so is cutting the chest open to bypass clogged arteries or amputating a leg.

If you are addicted to toxic food and have cravings that drive unhealthful eating, then you need to abstain from those triggers. The most effective way to beat the addictive drive is to engage in complete abstinence from addictive food. Abstinence keeps the "addiction motor" turned off. It is much easier to keep the motor turned off than to be constantly fighting addictive cravings and out-of-control appetites and mental obsessions.

HAVE A PLAN AND STICK TO IT

To get out and stay out of food addiction, one must always have a clearly defined and nonnegotiable plan, and then stick to it, no matter what. It takes vigilance and persistence at all times. One must not make compromises, or the addiction will take over again. The discipline of following a clearly defined plan *will* produce freedom!

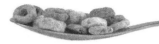

I like to compare getting out of food addiction to learning to ride a bike. A beginner may have some spills before he or she learns the proper balancing skill to ride a bike without falling. It may even take some reinforcement like a parent's helpful guidance, or a pair of training wheels attached to the bike. But eventually, with practice, one learns to ride without thinking about it anymore. Riding a bike becomes automatic, and then one is no longer focused on the learning process, but instead enjoys the pure pleasure of the scenic ride.

However, even the most seasoned cyclist must always be careful not to ride too fast on gravel, not to ride near the edge of pavement, and to pay close attention to busy intersections; otherwise, an accident could happen in a split second.

Likewise, it will always take careful planning and diligence to implement that plan, no matter how seasoned one is at eating healthfully.

BE PREPARED AT ALL TIMES

Plan ahead and always have food prepared in advance. Your health destiny is your responsibility, so be prepared at all times.

Unlike processed food dieting, no factory-prepared meals will be delivered to your doorstep. Keep your refrigerator well stocked with fresh vegetables, fruits, and soups for quick meals. Never wait until the refrigerator is empty to plan and prepare more food. Once you establish a routine of preparation, it will become second nature—but in the beginning, you may need to make this habit a top priority in order to develop it.

SLIP-UPS HAPPEN

Slip-ups, also known as lapses in judgment, happen from time to time—it's a part of transitioning into a whole new way of eating and living for the rest of one's life. Especially in the beginning, there's a learning curve and mistakes happen. I've had plenty of lapses in judgment. Even with cravings for the Standard American Diet completely gone, I've eaten as a result of being frustrated. I've eaten for stimulation because I was tired. I've eaten to regulate a mood. I've eaten for recreation with others when I wasn't a bit hungry. But most times, I've realized my error and moved on *quickly*.

However, relapse is the continual and intentional decision to compromise and cheat on a regular basis. These habitual compromises, even if they are seemingly insignificant at the time, *are* detrimental to freedom from food addiction. The willful decision to see how much one can cheat and get by; how much one can straddle the fence; or habitually overeat, and still keep food addiction eradicated from one's life is a next-to-impossible feat to accomplish.

With repetitive compromises, the addictive cravings can be ignited to full strength again. I've suffered from a relapse. It happens sometimes, even with the best of intentions. In order to have long-term freedom from food addiction, we must reach out to others for increased help and support if relapse happens—because to live in denial of the power of addiction is to remain its prisoner.

NEVER GIVE UP

Hard times happen. When life is turned upside down, it takes everything within you to muster the strength to keep going in the

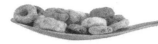

direction of health. But even when you have challenging days, stay committed to make wise food choices—as best as you can. There is never a valid excuse to quit. As Dr. Fuhrman states, "It will take strength, it will take effort, but the pleasures and rewards that you'll get from a healthy life will be priceless."

Please don't make the same mistake that I made and turn to low-nutrient food in times of great distress. It is *not* comfort food whatsoever, because it adds another layer of discomfort.

Instead, make a blended salad with a generous amount of prewashed greens, ground flaxseeds, almonds, and at least a cup of blueberries if you don't have the "oomph" to make anything else. Eating nutrient-rich food is the path to healing.

Looking back, many of my friends were offering to help me after my son's funeral. They would have been happy and willing to go to the store for me, or prepare green smoothies for me, or wash and cut up vegetables. But I refused their offers of help and paid a huge price for it.

Sometimes, the best gift we can give ourselves, and to others, is to reach out for help when we need it—and graciously receive that help—instead of succumbing to temptations in times of overwhelming distress.

I encourage anyone going through a hard time never to give up, no matter what. The sun *will* shine again, and happiness will return as one continues to stay the course. And in the meantime, reach out for help.

THE TRANSFORMATION ART EXHIBIT

From an early age, I wanted to be an artist when I grew up. In elementary school, I excelled at drawing and painting. To say that I had a paintbrush in my hand more than a pencil is no stretch of the imagination.

My parents had an old piano bench that was my art studio. That bench was filled with scraps of paper, watercolor paints, brushes, glue, scissors, glitter, pipe cleaners, cotton balls, and lots of crayons. Whenever I could, I would make something with my hands. My little art studio was my happy place, my comfort zone of escape from verbal and emotional abuse.

In my early teens, I painted a gigantic mural on the side of a large shed on my parents' farm. The shed faced a highly traveled road and received a lot of visibility. One by one, people would ask me to paint a mural for them.

As soon as I obtained my driver's license at age sixteen, I became a professional muralist. I painted murals throughout

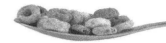

the region in churches, schools, homes, and businesses—in the midst of finishing high school and then going to college.

I further developed my drawing and painting skills at Purdue University; specifically, under the watchful eye and tutelage of Al Pounders, now professor emeritus of painting. He was tough, but he instilled in me the desire and passion to create significant works of art.

Years later, I traveled to Italy and Greece to study the Renaissance. While there, I got to see incredible masterpieces, including *The Creation of Adam* on the ceiling of the Sistine Chapel. I was profoundly impacted.

I wrote the following in my journal at the tomb of Michelangelo:

I am different now.

I don't know exactly how, but I am different.

My soul is at rest.

Undisturbed. Saturated.

Like film processing in a darkroom.

Silent. Hidden.

Like an unborn baby developing in a mother's womb.

Perhaps in the days and years to come the unveiling will occur.

May 2006

I came back from that trip changed. I had seen some of the best art eyes could ever behold. Yet, deep inside of me, I felt uncomfortably incongruent.

At that time, I was carrying a hundred pounds of excess weight. I thought, *Here I am, wanting to make significant works of art, yet desecrating the most significant masterpiece of all, my body.*

Something had to change, and I was ready to do whatever it would take.

In May 2008, I was in the middle of my friend Audrey Riley's art studio in Fort Wayne (I had met Audrey on that trip), when I had the following epiphany:

What would happen if I used food as an artistic medium? Just as a painter uses paint, or a sculptor uses metal, or a potter uses clay...to use food to make my body into the work of art that it was originally meant to be?

The idea seemed to me like divine inspiration. It was a catalyzing moment that lit a flame deep within me, and the clarity of vision was unstoppable.

Right there in Audrey's studio, an art exhibit was born—an exhibit that would use food as the artistic medium and my obese body as the point of departure. I would name it *Transformation.*

I knew instantly that I would follow Dr. Fuhrman's nutritional information as the impetus for change. Kurt and I had interacted with him via a phone consultation a few years earlier when we were seeking help for our son, who had just been diagnosed with Type I diabetes (juvenile diabetes). Out of desperation, I had Googled "reverse diabetes" and had discovered an article he had written on the topic.

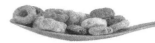

Basically, by eating whole, high-nutrient plant food, our son's diabetes could stabilize, and we would be able to reduce his insulin intake by half. But even more importantly, Dr. Fuhrman encouraged us that by eating this way, our son could have the best chance to live a fulfilling life, free of serious and life-threatening complications that eventually befall those with diabetes.

His logic made sense. *Everything* he said made sense, but we incorrectly assumed it would be too difficult to change our family's eating habits. We chose to go the conventional route instead, which was eating the typical Standard American Diet and injecting high doses of insulin to cover the surges of glucose. Our local pediatric endocrinologist (who specialized in treating kids with Type I diabetes) supported and promoted the conventional way—so that was the route we chose to go instead.

However, by that May of 2008, my blood pressure was dangerously high. I had been diagnosed with coronary artery disease and prediabetes, and I had numerous other maladies developing in and on my body, such as cracked heels, painful boils, and chronic low back pain.

I knew diets didn't work. I had tried every diet known on the planet, including weekly weight loss meetings, to no avail.

I knew I had an addiction to food—processed, sugary, salty, and high-fat foods—and I couldn't get free no matter what I did.

Thankfully, by this time *Eat to Live*, Dr. Fuhrman's classic work, was published. In it, he explained that, when the body is properly nourished, cravings for unhealthy foods dissipate, and then eventually go away.

I was all in.

I chose July 10, 2008, as the starting date for the art exhibit and created a rudimentary website to document it. I posted writings, pictures, and medical stats of my journey. I also posted a YouTube video of my changing body size set to music.

Little did I know that day of starting *Transformation*, that it would eventually inspire people from all over the world. I have received hundreds of notes throughout the years from people I have never met. For example, one day I received an email from a woman halfway around the globe. She wrote to tell me that one night, she was about to end her life by jumping off her high-rise apartment's balcony. However, as she was holding onto the railing, she felt compelled to go inside her apartment and read my online art exhibit. As she was reading it, hope filled her heart, and she wanted to live again. Afterward, she slept peacefully for the first time in months. Today, she is a happy mother of a preschooler and grateful to be alive.

Even though nearly a decade has passed since I started the art exhibit, I have left it online, and anyone can still visit it to be inspired and motivated. (www.EmilyBoller. com—*Transformation)*

The following are journal entries and a few pictures from it. I invite you to peruse my online art exhibit and view the many changing images that I posted on it—a picture is worth a thousand words—and be inspired and motivated by seeing what food can do for the body!

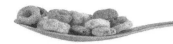

The Transformation Art Exhibit

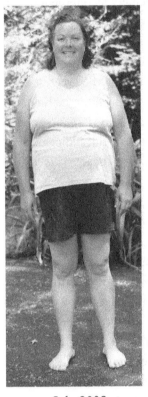 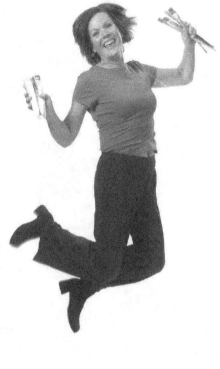

July 2008   July 2009

*"Every block of stone has a statue inside it
and it is the task of the sculptor to discover it."*

—*Michelangelo*

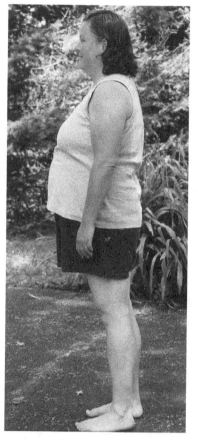

<u>PROLOGUE: JULY 3, 2008</u>

I am an artist, though an extremely incongruent one. It has been my passion to create significant works of art in my lifetime; yet, I have been desecrating the greatest work of art known to mankind, the human body. I am no good to the art world addicted, sick, or worse, dead. This addiction to mediocrity is about to change.

A week from today, July 10, 2008, I will embark on a journey of transformation. It will be the starting point I have chosen to begin to live again. Through this art exhibit, I want to address the issue of gluttony head-on; the violation, abuse, and desecration of a sacred masterpiece, the human body.

It is no longer my desire merely to make significant works of art; I also want to *be* a significant work of art.

My own obesity will be the point of departure from which this exhibit will evolve. What will happen to my body as I make wise food choices that support health? Will my art change as my body, health, and well-being transform? Will my own

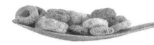

transformation inspire in the viewer a desire to change his or her life in some way also?

Just as a painter uses paint, or a sculptor uses metal, or a potter uses clay as mediums to form works of art, I will use food to transform my body into the work of art that it was originally designed to be.

I will be following the nutritional wisdom in Dr. Joel Fuhrman's book, *Eat to Live*, and will use food to transform my body into the work of art that it was originally designed to be. I have chosen to adhere to his guidelines, because most doctors merely want to control cardiovascular and obesity-related diseases with toxic drugs and surgery, and manage diabetes with medications and insulin; but he wants to eradicate these diseases altogether through excellent nutrition.

A PERFECT PROTOTYPE: JULY 10, 2008

Today, I am a perfect prototype of the American obesity epidemic. Unfortunately, I am the perfect, desecrated work of art designed to begin this creative journey.

For several years, I fluctuated between 225 and 235 pounds (height 5'8"), with my highest weight tipping the scale at 238 pounds; and at that same time, my highest waist circumference was fifty-one inches.

Obesity not only robs one of good health, but in general, overall quality of life. Unfortunately, it only takes a daily repetition of a few unwise choices to send one into the deep abyss of obesity; but, thankfully, there is a way out of the deadly disease!

STARVED TO OBESITY: AUGUST 10, 2008

I have eaten very well this past month. Prior to eating high-nutrient food, I was starving myself to obesity; I was consuming less than 500 points per day of nutrients based on the Aggregate Nutrient Density Index (ANDI) food scoring guide. Now I'm eating more than 3,000 points per day! I'm truly enjoying eating again, and my meals are free from calorie and exchange counting, weighing and measuring every morsel of food, and restrictive, chemical-laden diet food. My energy level is up, because my body is finally nourished for the first time in my life.

	One month ago	Today
Weight	226 pounds	206 pounds
Blood pressure	157 / 94	140 / 80
Waist	50"	45"
Fasting blood glucose	110	102
Total cholesterol	214	145
Triglycerides	203	101
HDL (good) cholesterol	47	43
Body Mass Index	35	31.5

It has only been one month of eating high-nutrient food, and I'm twenty pounds lighter! For the first time in my life, I get to enjoy *eating!*

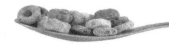

EXCITED: AUGUST 25, 2008

I'm excited today, because even throughout a season of intense personal stress, my blood pressure dropped to 118/69! This past March, during a time of low stress, my blood pressure was up to 157/94. That was one of those scary "reality checks" that triggered me to start doing something about changing my lifestyle.

I've been eating high-nutrient food for only six weeks now, and I'm feeling like a new person.

INCREMENTAL CHANGES: OCTOBER 10, 2008

Since I had repeatedly failed at trying to follow diets, I finally resigned myself to accept the many incremental changes I had to make in order to adjust to the burdensome handicap of obesity. Now, three months later, I realize how extremely misguided I was with those proven-to-fail diets, because my body was desperately craving nourishment! Below, you will see my numbers, which are improving each month, but what you won't be able to see are the vibrant colors and explosive cart-wheels of joyous freedom that I'm experiencing within!

	Before (July 10, 2008)	**Current** (October 10, 2008)
Weight	226 pounds	186 pounds
Blood pressure	157 / 94	112 / 70
Waist	50"	40"
BMI	35	28.3

Three months and 40 pounds lighter!
"The more you eat green the more you get lean."
—Joel Fuhrman, M.D.

AMAZED: NOVEMBER 10, 2008

I am amazed how well I feel these days. My blood pressure dropped further to 108/60, and I no longer have shortness of breath after climbing a flight of stairs. My weight loss slowed down this month, but I lost another inch around my waist.

Recently, I ate a small slice of cheesecake and felt miserable afterward. My favorite food now is a blueberry and spinach smoothie. My taste buds have changed, and I'm literally transforming into the work of art that I was originally meant to be.

TYPICAL HOLIDAY: DECEMBER 10, 2008

I've been displaying my stats and pictures since starting *Transformation* on July 10; and although I'm happy that my weight, blood pressure, BMI, cholesterol, and waist circumference have all dropped significantly, I'm most thrilled that now my body reacts to eating unhealthy food.

This past month, I ate what would be classified as a typical holiday indulgence for me: turkey, dinner rolls, butter, cheese, salad slathered in creamy dressing, pumpkin pie, Christmas cookies, and fudge. Several hours later, I got terribly sick (and that's putting it mildly).

The pain inside my gut felt like a continual stabbing of sharp knives. After my body naturally expelled its contents and broke into a feverish sweat, I immediately felt fine.

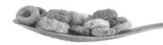

Dr. Fuhrman said that my body now reacts violently in order to protect itself when abused.

For many years, I had abused my body with unwise food choices on a daily basis and didn't even realize it. I had become accustomed to feeling blah...and didn't feel well unless I was eating the toxic food of the Standard American Diet: high-fat, high-salt, low-nutrient, processed food. I would experience fatigue, brain fog, and shakiness if I didn't eat right away.

Dr. Fuhrman calls this kind of addictive response "toxic hunger."

My body is now free from the addiction to toxic hunger!

I'm happy about numbers dropping, clothes fitting, joints not aching, and even feeling youthful again, but freedom from the addiction to toxic hunger, and the general malaise that goes along with it, are the results that I'm most excited about!

I've been rescued from chronic malnutrition that was leading me straight down a destructive path of unnecessary suffering and premature death.

	Before (July 10, 2008)	**Current** (December 10, 2008)
Weight	226 pounds	175 pounds
Blood Pressure	157/94	122/78
Waist	50"	38"
BMI	35	26.6

SIX MONTHS: JANUARY 10, 2009

Six months ago today, I embarked on the most life-changing adventure of my life, and six months from today, on July 10, 2009, I am confident that my blood tests will come back normal. Most importantly, I will have my health back!

By God's grace, diabetes, a nasty disease I hate with a passionate vengeance, will never be a part of my life. I am thrilled to have lost two more inches of cumbersome "belly fat" this past month; even through a couple of birthday celebrations, a major ice storm that knocked out the electrical power for several days and nights, Christmas and New Year's gatherings, and the many holiday traditions centered around high-fat, low-nutrient, processed food.

I'm at peace after years of striving. I have finally found a simple and economical way of eating for health that works, even through many unpredictable circumstances and changes.

	Before (July 10, 2008)	**Current** (January 10, 2009)
Weight	226 pounds	172 pounds
Blood pressure	157/94	96/60
Waist	50"	36"
BMI	35	26.1

FEBRUARY 1, 2009

Due to a major surgery to remove a benign tumor that I'm scheduled to have on February 9th, and recovery time afterward, I will not be posting progress updates until April 10, 2009. Thank

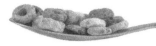

for your patient understanding. I will be preparing and freezing blueberry and spinach smoothies, vegetable soup, and lentil stew so that I will be able to have plenty of nourishing food stocked up for the journey ahead.

SURGERY RECOVERY UPDATE: FEBRUARY 23, 2009

I'm posting before April 10 to give a brief recovery update. I am grateful the surgery went well, and I'm glad it's over! The surgeon removed a tumor that was the size of a cantaloupe, and I lost five or six pounds instantly. (But it wasn't any fun!) I'm

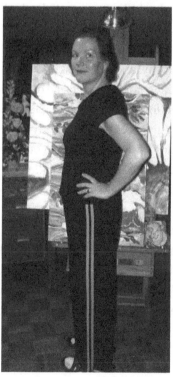

getting stronger each day, and I'm very thankful that I was relatively healthy going into surgery...another reason to eat for health; one never knows when an unexpected surgery may occur. My fasting blood sugar is now 85; way in the safe range for being nondiabetic. Considering I was prediabetic in July, I'm doing cartwheels just thinking about not needing to prick my finger or give myself a shot of insulin every time I eat! (Not to mention the heavy financial burden, rise in insurance costs, and serious complications and suffering as a result.)

APRIL 3, 2009

I won't have access to my computer to post updates on April 10, so I'll post some basic stats today. My waist circumference is 34" (down from 50" in July), BMI is 23.7 (down from 35), weight is 153 pounds (down from 226 pounds), fasting blood sugar is 85, and my recent blood pressure was 92/57. My blood pressure was 157/94 a year ago! I no longer wear plus size 22, and I now fit into size 10 pants with much ease.

CARTWHEELS: JUNE 29, 2009

Greetings to all! If I could do back flips and cartwheels, I would post a video of me doing them today! Know that I am silently screaming with great joy and excitement right now!

My family doctor noticed that my abdominal skin, after I lost so much belly fat, retracted back to normal, which he doesn't typically observe with patients who lose a lot of weight. He also commented that I've taken at least fifteen years off my age. Thank you, greens, beans, fruits, nuts, and seeds! Thank you, Dr. Fuhrman, for blazing the trail to get America's health back! Food really is an artistic medium to restore the body to its original design and function.

A well-nourished body truly is a work of art.

	Before (July 10, 2008)	After (July 10, 2009)
Weight	226 pounds	139 pounds
Blood pressure	157/94	110/68
Waist	50"	31"
Fasting blood glucose	110	80

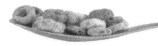

Hemoglobin A1C	Prediabetic	5.3
Total cholesterol	214	157
Triglycerides	203	68
LDL (bad) cholesterol	126	87
HDL (good) cholesterol	47	56
BMI	35	21.5

The following maladies are gone: coronary artery disease, hypertension, prediabetes, angina, shortness of breath, chronic fatigue, painful boils, cracked heels, and low back pain.

These nuisances are also gone: snoring, bloated abdo-men, puffy fingers and face, a buffalo hump of fat on my back at the base of my neck, stiff and achy joints, immobility, and brain fog.

EPILOGUE

Soon after these photos were taken, I celebrated my weight loss journey by going on a bike ride. Not using the best of caution, I zoomed down a hilly, gravel road. My front tire lost control in the loose stones, and my body hit the road at full force.

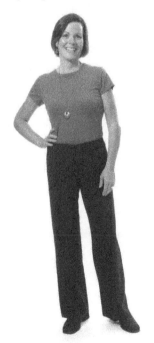

Photo credit: Jeff Crane

I had to get X-rays, and as I was lying flat on my back under the machine, I overheard the technician instruct his assistant to reposition my body because I was *thin!*

That four-letter word was music to this woman's ears; the perfect ending to an adventuresome year of transformation!

The human body certainly can become the significant work of art that it was originally designed to be.

"Only in excellent physical and emotional health can a person's full potential be realized. Emily Boller is a true artist whose inner beauty of spirit was trapped inside her by the shackles of her food addictions, now set free. I am very proud of her."

—Joel Fuhrman, M.D.

FREQUENTLY ASKED QUESTIONS

WHERE DO YOU GET YOUR PROTEIN AND CALCIUM?

As long as you are eating a variety of different plant foods, your body *will* get plenty of essential amino acids and calcium to sustain life and thrive.

Green vegetables, nuts, seeds, and beans are rich in protein. Green vegetables have the most protein per calorie of all. For instance, broccoli has about twice as much protein as steak![44]

Animal proteins increase the production of a hormone called IGF-1 (insulin-like growth factor). Much of this hormone is associated with aging and the increased growth of cancer cells.[45]

If you are worried about calcium, studies show fruits and vegetables are protective against osteoporosis (bone density loss). Substances such as animal products, salt, caffeine, refined sugar, alcohol, nicotine, antacids, antibiotics, steroids, thyroid

---

44   Fuhrman, *Eat to Live*, 142.
45   Fuhrman, *The End of Dieting*, 137.

hormone, and vitamin A supplements actually induce calcium loss in the urine.[46]

All green vegetables are high in calcium. Plus, they have higher absorption rates than dairy products. Not to mention that cruciferous vegetables, such as broccoli, cauliflower, kale, collards, and various cabbages have sulfur-containing chemicals (isothiocyanates) that inhibit cancer-causing substances (carcinogens). They actually inhibit the growth of carcinogens and induce cancer cell death![47]

That food pyramid that you may have memorized in high school health or home economics was incorrect. If you want to understand the phenomenal science behind all of this, study Dr. Fuhrman's books and articles for yourself. Our bodies are fascinating machines that were designed to be fueled by plants.

DO YOU EAT OUT?

Yes, but I didn't in the beginning.

I do not recommend eating out until you have established at least a solid month or two of sobriety. It takes at least that much time for the taste buds to change and for you to get "out of the woods" with toxic hunger—with the worst being the first week.

After cravings have subsided, and you have established clearly defined boundary lines, then it may be possible to venture out again, depending on the severity of entanglements you were trapped in. But don't rush it. It is not worth slipping back into addiction during one meal.

---

46   Fuhrman, *Eat to Live,* 103–107.
47   Fuhrman, *Super Immunity*, 251.

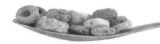

I lived most of my life trapped in food addiction. Then I got free, and then I relapsed into it again. I will do *anything*—whatever it takes—to remain free. It only takes one bite of an addictive food to begin to unravel progress. It's just not worth it.

Many times, I drink a green smoothie beforehand and order a salad and/or steamed vegetables at the restaurant. Afterward, I eat the remainder of the meal at home or in the car. (Insulated coolers are a nutritarian's best friend!) Also, roasted edamame beans can be purchased online, or you can make your own roasted chickpeas—there are many recipes nowadays. Put the roasted beans in a plastic bag and tuck it inside your purse to take to the restaurant. No one cares, because getting together is about building relationships. Furthermore, it is no one's business what you do or do not eat to stay healthy. If you don't make a big deal about it, nobody else will, either—unless you hang around rude people. Fast food restaurants, such as Subway, have salads, and they have a nice selection of veggies to add as well. Pizza Hut, Golden Corral, Whole Foods Markets and various other eating establishments have salad bars, which work well too.

A good steakhouse usually has excellent salads, and if you go early enough—not at the rush hour—they are willing to be creative with their vegetables, including steaming them. However, make it clear that you do not want salt, butter, or oil. My favorite restaurant has a steamed vegetable platter for an appetizer. They are very good about omitting the salt and sauces per my request.

Someone from Dr. Fuhrman's member center printed simple dietary instructions on business cards to give to wait staff and chefs. Those cards have been a very successful tool for her.

Another member, whose husband travels overseas on business trips, packs an extra piece of luggage with healthy food for her husband. She packs the food in dry ice until her husband arrives at his destination and can refrigerate it. It may sound burdensome, but he lost nearly a hundred pounds in less than a year. Today, he is living in optimal health and fitness, is off his CPAP machine (for snoring), and takes no medications!

An elderly gentleman whom I interviewed for "Disease Proof" (in his eighties and running marathons!) goes on a lot of cruises with his wife. He works with the wait staff beforehand, and they have always been happy to accommodate his dietary needs.

If nothing else, you can always have a green smoothie before leaving home, and then order a small salad and herbal tea at the restaurant. The meal should be about sharing relationships with friends; not food.

I meet my close friends for walks and talks on the many fitness trails in the area—and we all enjoy them so much. A brisk walk with a friend is invigorating!

DO YOU EXERCISE?

Dr. Fuhrman says that exercise is not optional.

Experts are now calling a sedentary lifestyle the "new smoking."

If you are in the habit of sitting all day, it is time to get moving—even if it is just a short walk—do *something*.

The year I lost a hundred pounds, I started walking a half-hour before breakfast and then a half-hour before my evening

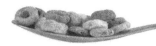

meal, because I was prediabetic. Walking prior to a meal was similar to taking oral diabetes medications or insulin. It was a natural way to control high glucose levels in my bloodstream, thus enhancing weight loss. It wasn't a brisk walk, but it was enough to get my body moving.

After I lost forty pounds, I felt well enough to substitute my morning walk with working out on an elliptical machine at the Y. Then I started lifting free weights and using a StairMaster. Through the course of that year, I was able to increase my endurance and strength incrementally. I had toned up muscles that I hadn't used since my teenage years.

Fourteen months later, I ran my first four-mile race since high school, and I felt exuberant! There are many benefits to exercise. Besides helping with weight loss and blood sugar control, it is a natural antidepressant when used alongside a nutritarian diet. Daily exercise is an important component to getting out and staying out of food addiction.

Plus, as we age, we lose muscle mass, and exercise helps build muscle. We need strong muscles to protect our bones in our elderly years. In fact, Dr. Fuhrman says that women who engage in regular exercise are twice as likely to avoid hip fractures later in life. Staying fit protects against injuries.

Recently, I have discovered a fitness video produced by Leslie Sansone called "Walk Away the Pounds," and her workouts challenge just about every muscle in the body. When I am finished with one of her workouts, I feel like I truly did work every muscle in my body.

Movement of any kind conditions muscles, not to mention that it boosts serotonin levels in the brain and lifts moods. Dr.

Fuhrman says that regular exercise is better than an antidepressant—and without the adverse side effects. Find something you enjoy doing, and then get moving. You will feel alive and well when you do![48]

DO YOU WEIGH, MEASURE, OR COUNT QUANTITIES?

Dr. Fuhrman says to forget about counting calories. He also repeatedly states that the nutritarian diet-style is not about eating less food—it is about the nutritional *quality* of food one eats. "It isn't how much you eat that determines your weight; it's what you eat."[49] He also adds, "You don't have to weigh portions and count calories because a bigger portion of these particular foods is better than a smaller one. Instead of eating less food, then, eat three substantially sized meals a day—of the right kinds of food."[50] "Remember, if it's a vegetable with the color of green, it is rich in micronutrients and low in calories. It's a green light to eat more of it. The more greens you eat, the increased likelihood you will eat less of something else that is higher in calories."[51]

In addition, many of the fibrous, raw vegetables take more calories to chew, digest, and assimilate than the calories they provide. And, as previously stated, when cruciferous vegetables (cabbage, kale, broccoli, cauliflower, collards) are consumed,

---

48   Joel Fuhrman, M.D., *Treating Depression Naturally*.
     https://www.drfuhrman.com/library/position-papers/2/
     treating-depression-naturally
49   Fuhrman, *The End of Dieting,* 8.
50   Ibid, 87.
51   Ibid, 126.

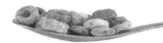

they boost the immune system and kill cancer cells.[52] Mushrooms and onions also boost the immune system and fight cancer; not to mention that greens, mushrooms, and onions inhibit the growth of new blood vessels that fuel fat. They actually *facilitate* fat loss![53]

The only foods that should be carefully monitored are nuts and seeds. Dr. Fuhrman recommends limiting nuts and seeds to one ounce per day for women and two ounces per day for men *if you have weight to lose* (in addition to one tablespoon of ground flaxseeds per day). When the excess weight is off, these amounts can be adjusted to higher amounts, if desired. However, don't skip the nuts and seeds because not only do they suppress appetite and pull bad fats out of the body,[54] they also are loaded with important Omega-3 fatty acids that protect against depression, heart disease, and cancer.[55]

I have a digital food scale. I weigh one ounce of nuts every morning and then set them aside in a small bowl to be eaten later in the day. Doing that is a clearly defined boundary line for me that I do not cross. If I don't carefully monitor nuts and seeds, I can easily overeat them and gain weight. (Some folks have found measuring *all* food at each meal to be beneficial for them in order to establish healthy boundaries—at least in the

---

52   Fuhrman, *Super Immunity,* 67–70.
53   Joel Fuhrman, M.D., "Super Immunity—Win the War on Cancer." Dr. Fuhrman's Health Immersion, October 2012, the Dolce Resort, Basking Ridge, New Jersey.
54   Fuhrman, *The End of Dieting,* 118.
55   Joel Fuhrman, M.D., *Super Immunity*, (New York: HarperCollinsPublishers, 2011), 118.

beginning—after years of unrestrained eating. If that works the best for you, do whatever *you* may need to do to be free from destructive habits.)

A goal Dr. Fuhrman often gives is to shoot for a whole pound of raw vegetables a day, one pound of cooked vegetables, one cup of beans, one tablespoon of flaxseeds, one ounce of raw nuts/seeds (two ounces for men), and three to four fresh fruits—but you don't have to be rigid about it if that is too much food for you to eat. In addition, you may eat one cup of cooked, starchy vegetables or whole grains; two ounces of avocado; and two tablespoons of dried fruit such as raisins (optional). All this high-fiber, nutrient-rich plant food then suppresses the appetite and aids in controlling emotional and addictive eating.[56]

It is also very important to eat only three meals or fewer per day—and to go to bed on a completely empty stomach. When snacking between meals is eliminated, the body is able to rest from digesting food nonstop. It is helpful to know that a growling stomach is merely a signal that digestion has ended. Period. It doesn't mean you need to eat again! If you've been eating a steady diet of toxic food, you may experience uncomfortable physical symptoms when you stop snacking between meals. (This toxic withdrawal is explained in Chapter Two.) However, it's important to remember that these symptoms will eventually go away as you consistently eat only nutrient-rich food. In addition, the extended time of fasting from dinnertime to breakfast the next morning gives the body a much-needed rest.

---

56   Fuhrman, *Eat to Live*, 29.

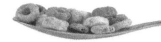

This enables it to focus its energy on detoxification, healing and repairing—which is vital to optimal health and well-being.[57]

IS THE NUTRITARIAN DIET-STYLE COSTLY?

The beautiful thing about the nutritarian diet-style is that it can be done successfully on a shoestring budget and still be just as effective as a gourmet, high-end version. My daughter budgeted sixty dollars per week for nutritarian meals that she made in her apartment when she was in college. For others, a hundred dollars per week is not enough.

I eat this way for about eighty dollars per week. However, when I was overeating habitually on the Standard American Diet, I was consuming at least a hundred and fifty dollars' worth of food and beverages every week. (Plus, it takes more calories to fuel an overweight body.) I save at least seventy-five dollars every week now, as compared to my former lifestyle. That is a savings of more than $3,000 a year! That is harsh and hard to admit, but it is the truth.

In addition, I no longer need to visit an endocrinologist or a cardiologist, or need expensive lab tests, surgical procedures, hospitalizations, or medications. (Heart bypass surgery alone can cost more than $115,000!) And due to a strong immune system now, I haven't had bronchitis in more than ten years. Prior to eating this way, every winter since my early twenties, I would catch a cold that would develop into a nasty case of bronchitis. Between doctor visits, prescription meds, and over-the-counter drugs to help alleviate the symptoms, it was *not* a cheap illness.

---

57 Fuhrman, *The End of Dieting*, 23–24.

None of us can afford to be addicted to the Standard American Diet. It not only robs and destroys health—but finances as well. Making a commitment to the nutritarian diet-style is cost-*effective*!

NOTES FROM THE HEART

A NOTE TO PARENTS AND PARENTS-TO-BE

We live in a culture inundated with sweets and junk food everywhere we turn. We can't get away from it. Food is not the problem; the Standard American Diet is.

Let me tell you about a time I learned an important lesson about this very toxic diet. I fed my children fast food kids' meals, processed cereals, crackers, chips, ice cream novelties, chicken nuggets, deli meats, hot dogs, macaroni and cheese, TV dinners, frozen pot pies, and pizza pockets. Such convenience food was standard fare for young mothers of the '80s and '90s.

I did provide their bodies with carrots, celery, lettuce, green beans, broccoli, and apples; but the mainstay food was "home cooked meals" of the Standard American Diet: spaghetti and garlic bread, meatloaf and scalloped potatoes, homemade pepperoni pizza, grilled chicken and baked potatoes with butter, pot roast and biscuits, cornbread and milk, beef and noodles.

If I could unwind the clock for a do-over, I certainly would. My son Daniel, who was diagnosed with Type I diabetes at age eleven, died, in part, due to a toxic food overdose.

Starting at age fifteen, if his blood sugars would go high, the avalanche of brain-damaging glucose spikes would create a medical delirium (metabolic encephalopathy) with symptoms of psychosis. The hallucinations and delusions, combined with the adverse side effects of some of the mind-altering medications he was put on, would then negatively affect *everyone* in his path, including himself. As long as he kept his blood sugars stable, his mind would remain stable and he could manage the challenges of life. Unfortunately, he lived in a culture inundated with fast food everywhere he went—and it took every ounce of his energy to remain free from the temptations and peer pressure to succumb to them.

Before his funeral, I found his trash can filled with empty boxes of processed cereals, empty jars of honey-roasted peanut butter, empty packages of cookies, and empty bottles of sodas. In his car were crumpled-up sacks and food wrappers from three different fast food restaurants. When I reviewed his blood glucose meter history, I discovered his blood sugars were continually more than 350 the week leading up to his death.

Food addiction, causing the glucose spikes and delirium, contributed to his death by suicide.

Junk food and fast food are rampant across America; those addicted to this toxic diet are eating themselves to death. True, drug addiction kills, but Dr. Fuhrman says that food addiction kills so many more. Obesity alone kills more than 300,000 people a year.

Sure, we may have a hereditary propensity to develop obesity, heart disease, diabetes, cancer—that is the loaded gun

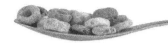

we may have been given due to our family genes—but it's our dietary choices that determine if we pull the trigger or not.

Unfortunately, rearing children on the Standard American Diet sets the stage for a potential lifetime of food addiction, mental struggles, and nutritional diseases—and it begins even before conception. "According to studies, our diet, not just during pregnancy but even before conception, has profound effects in determining the health, intelligence, and immune systems of our children."[58]

In Dr. Fuhrman's book *Disease-Proof Your Child,* he states: "We parents have a huge responsibility and can help guide and shape our offspring into healthy and happy adults, or, through abuse, neglect, ignorance, and even convenience, we can damage their future. We know with certainty that the foods we feed our kids during childhood play a large role in dictating their future health."[59]

For example, according to Caldwell Esselstyn, M.D., the foundation of coronary artery disease is firmly established by the end of high school here in the United States. Based on autopsies performed in 1999 on young adults between the ages of seventeen and thirty-four who died from accidents, suicides, and homicides, coronary artery disease was already widespread in this age group.[60]

---

58 Fuhrman, *Fast Food Genocide,* 2.

59 Joel Fuhrman, M.D., *Disease Proof Your Child,* (New York: St. Martin's Press, 2005), 104.

60 Caldwell B. Esselstyn, Jr., M.D., "A plant-based diet and coronary artery disease: a mandate for effective therapy," *Journal of Geriatric Cardiology,* accessed May 3, 2018, https://www.ncbi.nlm.nih.gov/pmc/articles/PMC5466936/

Set the example by demonstrating living in optimal health yourself. Stock your kitchen with a variety of delicious food and make mealtimes a pleasurable and peaceful experience for all. If you need motivation and ideas for making kid-friendly, high-nutrient meals, Dr. Fuhrman and his wife, Lisa, who have reared four children together, have shared those recipes in *Disease-Proof Your Child*.

If you are a "foodie"—one who is particularly interested in food experiences and recipes as a pleasurable hobby—be mindful of children's health needs in the process. Consider directing your hobby's focus toward perfecting great-tasting recipes that promote health and well-being. The internet is loaded with nutritarian recipes now.

Parents also have a substantial role in preventing disordered eating in their children's lives by providing healthy and great-tasting food choices at home. Excessive control, such as putting children on restrictive diets, sets the stage for developing negative perceptions toward food. "When a parent attempts to control his or her child's eating, a child may then try to regain self control of eating by not eating other food or starting to binge eat."[61] In other words, have the great-tasting, high-nutrient food available to select from, but allow the child to honor his or her own fullness and satiety cues. This will prevent negative perceptions toward food.

61　"Parents Perception Towards Food Can Influence Child's Eating Habits," *Eating Disorder Hope,* October 12, 2013, accessed May 2, 2018, https://www.eatingdisorderhope.com/blog/parents-pressure-of-children-eating-habits-may-create-eating-disorders.

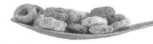

And whatever you do, please don't make a big deal out of a number on a scale. Both praise and shame have the potential to negatively impact a child who may have a genetic predisposition for an eating disorder. Self-worth cannot be measured by a number on a scale or a clothing size. Praise your child in other areas of his or her life that are totally unrelated to physical appearances. And do not call yourself or others "fat." It may be an accurate description of being overweight, but it is similar to calling a person who struggles with mental illness "psycho," or a person with cognitive challenges "retarded." Derogatory names wound young, impressionable minds and hearts, potentially causing them to develop to a negative self-image, which can foster eating disorders.

In addition, if you think your child may have a susceptibility for eating disorders, be aware of his or her exposure to high-risk activities that encourage a child to maintain a certain body size: ballet, gymnastics, fashion modeling, figure skating, cheerleading, wrestling, to name a few. (This may also include activities that emphasize heavy exercise, such as long-distance running.) "Dieting and a high-risk activity combined with a genetic vulnerability could send an individual into a full-fledged eating disorder."[62]

Be aware of your children's behaviors. Many times, children cannot clearly articulate pain as a result of abuse, and/or emotional and psychological trauma—but there are signs. If you are unsure, please seek the help of a professional counselor.

---

62   Jenni Schaefer, *Goodbye Ed, Hello Me,* (McGraw-Hill Education, 2009), 35.

Nothing is foolproof, of course, but being aware enough to take the necessary steps to prevent eating disorders from developing in the first place is a precious gift you can give to your children.

A NOTE TO COMMUNITIES OF FAITH

Throughout those years that I worked for Dr. Fuhrman, I met and interviewed multitudes of people from all over the country who had eradicated their food addictions and restored their health simply by changing the food they put into their mouths. I discovered that what a person ingests is important to every aspect of life. However, there is no place in the Bible that says, "Thou shalt not eat doughnuts."

Nevertheless, gluttony is mentioned several times in Scriptures, and it is a serious matter.

According to Merriam-Webster, gluttony is excessive indulgence. This self-destructive eating fuels obesity and disease. According to Roland Sturm, Ph.D., senior economist and professor of policy analysis at RAND Graduate School, obesity *outranks* smoking and drinking alcohol in disease, adverse consequences, and health care costs. Nevertheless, smoking and drinking have received more consistent attention in recent decades in both clinical practice and public health policy.[63] Furthermore, in *The End of Dieting,* Dr. Fuhrman states, "In

---

63   Roland Sturm, "The Effects of Obesity, Smoking, and Drinking on Medical Problems and Costs," accessed May 4, 2018. https://www.ncbi.nlm.nih.gov/pubmed/11900166.

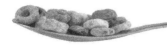

a matter of years, excess body weight is projected to overtake smoking as the primary cause of death in the United States."[64]

I was raised in a church culture that taught abstinence from drinking alcohol, using illegal drugs, and smoking cigarettes— and my parents reinforced it at home. Today, many communities of faith adhere to this same incongruent position regarding smoking and drinking, while fully condoning gluttony.

In 2009, six months after starting my journey to earn back my health, I did an experiment. I wanted to see what it would feel like to purchase a pack of cigarettes at a local gas station... at nearly fifty years old! (I had a lifetime of indoctrination built into my psyche concerning the harmful effects of alcohol, illegal drugs, and nicotine—of which I am eternally grateful for —because I was spared potentially developing addictions to those substances.)

So, I walked into the gas station and nervously looked around to make sure I didn't know anyone. When I stepped up to the counter to ask for a pack, I didn't even know what brand to ask for. I mumbled the name of a brand, not even knowing if it was a common one a female my age would buy or not. I glanced over my shoulder to make sure no one recognized me. My heart was pounding.

When the clerk retrieved the pack and rang it up at the register, I couldn't believe what it cost! Suddenly, I found myself handing over money for something that I knew was totally self-destructive. I felt very ashamed, and I would have felt even more embarrassed if someone I knew had witnessed the transaction.

---

64   Fuhrman, *The End of Dieting*, 4.

After throwing the spare change and cigarettes into my purse as quickly as possible, I dashed out of there.

Every fiber of my being knew that spending money on a self-destructive substance was wrong; yet, throughout my entire life, I didn't blink an eye at spending even one penny on self-destructive food, such as candy bars, chips, curly fries, shakes, doughnuts, and the like. My experiment enlightened me. The values we are taught at a young age, which are then reinforced in adulthood, greatly influence our behaviors.

For whatever reason, teaching on the harmful effects of the Standard American Diet has been overlooked by many churches. Doughnuts and pastries are still a valuable addition to Sunday morning gatherings. But hopefully, that will be changing soon.

Dr. Michael Klaper, a physician in nutrition-based medicine, describes what happens within minutes of eating sugar:

Within minutes, your bloodstream is flooded with sugar. Soon the structural proteins in all your tissues—the elastic fibers of your skin, the hemoglobin in your blood, the filter membranes in your kidneys, the inner lining of your blood vessels, the lenses of your eyes—all get 'sticky' with sugar (the chemists say they become 'glycosylated.') In the 98.6 F metabolic 'oven' of our body, the sugars and proteins melt together and oxidize, like the browning of bread crust (called the 'Maillard reaction.')

These oxidized, damaged, and congealed proteins, officially called 'Advanced Glycation End Products' do not function normally—the gummed-up, oxidized protein

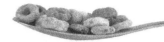
fibers break, skin cracks in the sunlight, eyes become less permeable to light, muscled proteins do not contract as vigorously, brain function dwindles—sound familiar?[65]

Years ago, I heard a local law enforcement officer speak at a meeting for young people. He told them that most car accidents at night were related to alcohol, and many car accidents in the morning were caused by blood sugar issues. Eating that sweet pastry early in the morning can influence the brain's ability to concentrate and function properly.

The detrimental effects that self-destructive eating can have on a person's life are profound. Today, in the U.S. alone, more than a hundred million people are living with diabetes or prediabetes, according to the Centers for Disease Control.[66] In addition, heart disease is the leading cause of death for both men and women in the U.S.[67] "Dietary ignorance, coupled with the addictive nature of refined foods, is now the leading cause of premature death in the modern world."[68]

Diseases of the Standard American Diet are literally killing us!

---

65   Michael Klaper, M.D., "Slaying the Sugary Beast," DoctorKlaper.com, December 19, 2014, accessed April 20, 2018, http://doctorklaper.com/answers/answers15/

66   Centers for Disease Control and Prevention, "New CDC report: More than 100 million Americans have diabetes or prediabetes," assessed May 9, 2018, https://www.cdc.gov/media/releases/2017/p0718-diabetes-report.html.

67   Centers for Disease Control and Prevention, "Heart Disease Facts," assessed May 9, 2018, https://www.cdc.gov/heartdisease/facts.htm.

68   Fuhrman, *The End of Dieting,* 43.

The late Rev. Leonard Ravenhill stated years ago that gluttony was the acceptable sin of the American Church. However, it has been my experience that gluttony is now the *promoted* sin of the American Church.

According to Dr. Fuhrman, the ten most dangerous foods are:

1. Smoked, barbecued, or conventionally raised red meat

2. Commercial baked goods

3. Butter

4. Pancakes and doughnuts

5. Soda (including sugar-free sodas)

6. Fried food

7. Highly salted food

8. Hot dogs and luncheon meats

9. White sugar (and maple syrup, honey, agave)

10. Sweetened dairy products[69]

Dr. Fuhrman also says that children, especially, are more susceptible to the destructive influences of such food, because growing and dividing cells are at greater risk when exposed to toxic compounds. In other words, this unhealthy diet can do more damage to a young body than to an adult one. Children's vulnerable cells become dysplastic (a precancerous condition) and, over the years, turn cancerous. In adulthood, the cancer becomes detectable.[70]

---

69   Joel Fuhrman, M.D., "Dr. Fuhrman's Guide to the Ten Best and Worst Foods," *Dr. Fuhrman.com,* accessed May 1, 2018, http://info.drfuhrman.com/10-best-10-worst-foods-for-longevity.

70   Fuhrman, *Disease-Proof Your Child,* 79–83.

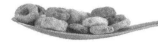

Additionally, Dr. Robert Lustig, pediatric endocrinologist and professor of pediatrics in the Division of Endocrinology at the University of California-San Francisco, states that sugar drives metabolic disease and is the alcohol of the child. Children are getting *diseases of alcohol*—without alcohol.[71]

Perhaps it's time for all of us to get the doughnuts out of our Sunday school classrooms and fellowship halls...and sugary snacks and diet sodas out of our Bible study gatherings.

May it not be said of houses of worship that they are modern-day crack houses, making provision for self-destructive entanglements. Instead, may they be sanctuaries of refuge from the onslaught of unhealthy temptations that promote addiction and disease.

It is time for all of us to rise up and live in freedom from food addiction—so that we can live in optimal health and fulfill our callings and destinies. It is also time to bless our children's futures, not create stumbling blocks and addictions that may take them a lifetime to overcome.

The Lord's best plans for all of us are for good; not obesity, heart disease, hypertension, cancer, diabetes, fatigue, dementia, depression, food addiction, and a myriad of other afflictions. We can no longer flirt with self-destructive indulgences, because the devil is having a heyday watching us become sick, lethargic, and barely functioning.

---

71   Interview by Jay Vera, "Dr. Lustig: Type 2 Diabetes is 'Processed Food Disease,'" *Crossfit; The Journal*, March 22, 2017, accessed May 3, 2018, https://journal.crossfit.com/article/cfj-lustig-rorary-interview.

Communities of faith have the awesome potential to be safe places where individuals can be set free from addictions. The very nature of their function allows them to help those trapped in entanglements.

Perhaps in the past we didn't know any better, but now that we know the truth, let's consider being sanctuaries that promote health and healing instead of disease and destruction.

It truly is time for change.

A NOTE FOR TEACHERS AND FUNDRAISERS

The following note was written by an older gentleman on Dr. Fuhrman's member center. He gave me permission to share it:

When I was 12 years old, I had to sell chocolate candy bars for our Catholic school. The candy bars were big. They measured two inches wide x one inch thick x eight inches long. I thought, I could sell a lot of them. So, I took about six boxes with twelve candy bars in each box. However, I could only sell two boxes. I had four boxes left, so I eventually ate all forty-eight candy bars! Then I would think, What am I going to do? Where will I get the money to pay for all of the candy bars that I have eaten? I ended up stealing money from my mother to pay for them. To this day I am ashamed of this horrible episode in my life. I still remember it as if it happened yesterday–and it happened more than fifty-five years ago! What were those nuns thinking by giving us all that candy to take home to sell?

—Peter Taurino

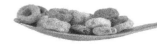

A DAUGHTER'S NOTE

Another member, Angela, shared the following:

I have never really thought of the cause of my father's death to be food addiction, but I now realize that my father died from food addiction. He was a physician and was diagnosed with Type 2 diabetes when he was 37 years old. After years of using medications to treat his symptoms (eleven of them), while buying candy and pastries in bulk from Costco, he died at the ripe age of 64. I now understand this was addictive behavior, because he knew that changing his diet would make his symptoms go away. He knew what the consequences of his behavior would be, yet he kept gorging on unhealthy food for 25 years...25 years of hospital stays and all sorts of nasty diabetic side effects. He was not a dummy, yet he engaged in this irrational behavior.

—Angela Biggar

MY OLDEST DAUGHTER'S PERSPECTIVE

One day, I asked my oldest daughter if she could write down what the addiction was like for her when I was trapped in it. (Oftentimes, it is easy to surround ourselves in a cloak of denial that our food choices don't affect others, but they do.) This was her response:

My mom's food addiction was a source of tension at times, especially if she was on a new diet. I could see the ups and downs with her struggle to lose weight and the fight not to give into food cravings. She would go through a phase of excitement from trying a new diet, but it was always short-lived. After seeing little to no results, she'd get discouraged and depressed and go to food for comfort and escape again."

—*Ruth Yaroslaski*

WISE WORDS FROM MY MOTHER

At age eighty-six, my mother suffered a stroke. After she was discharged from a six-week stay in rehab, Dr. Fuhrman's *3 Steps to Incredible Health* presentation was on the local PBS station. She watched it with great interest and decided to change her eating habits that day.

Even though she was moderately incapacitated from the stroke—over the next year, she lost eighty pounds, got off insulin that she had been taking for more than twenty years, lowered her dangerously high blood pressure, and gained enough strength to be relatively mobile again. I was very proud of her accomplishments, even in the midst of the hurdles and challenges she faced each day.

Prior to that show, she incorrectly assumed that she was too old to change or see improvements in her health and well-being. To her complete surprise, she learned that it is never too late to change.

She got to live four more years and meet her first great-grandchild. I wrote the following words down before her eventual passing:

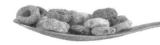

Health first…everything else second. One's health should come first above all other priorities; otherwise, other things will crowd it out. My main occupation now is making time for my food preparation, daily exercises, and adequate rest. If you are young, don't wait until you are old to change your priorities and eating habits. If you are old, it's never too late to change and get healthier. Don't cheat yourself out of the best health that's possible. Where there is a will—there is always a way.

—Helen Taylor

A NOTE FROM MY HUSBAND

Emily and I were young and clueless before we got married. When she told me she had a "problem" with food, I thought, *Everyone eats an extra piece of cake now and then; it's no big deal.* But I didn't realize how big of an issue it was until after we got married. It was difficult to watch Emily suffer with such a severe food addiction and ongoing eating disorder that drained the life out of her. I felt helpless, hopeless, and angry at times. It took years of trial and error finally to realize that I couldn't change her. I could only change myself.

If you have someone you love who is struggling with yo-yo dieting, a controlling food addiction, or any eating entanglement, there is hope for both of you. There is a way through it to the other side, but it will take time, patience, and unconditional love to get there.

I share the following tips, not as an expert on the topic, but as someone who has learned the hard way what works:

- Be honest with yourself and acknowledge your feelings. Stuffing your frustrations and anger will only make it worse–and then eventually you may explode in unhealthy ways.

- Be committed to the relationship.

- Realize you can't change others. The only person that you can change is yourself.

- There may be times when you'll need to pull back so your "boat" doesn't sink. A person drowning in addiction can pull others down with him or her, so maintain your own mental, spiritual, emotional, and physical health; just don't abandon your loved one.

- Seek professional counseling for your loved one as well as yourself. Not all counselors are equal. If a counselor isn't helpful, then keep looking until you find a good fit. The key is being willing to be totally honest about the underlying root problems that psychologically and emotionally fuel addiction.

- Don't quit. Never give up. Never give in. Never, never, never. In the words of Emily's great-aunt Mabel, "When you reach the end of your rope, tie a knot and hang on!"

—Kurt Boller

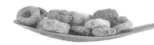

A FINAL NOTE

The last Christmas season before my son Daniel died, his church gave a "care package" of Christmas cookies to each college student. In order not to be rude, he graciously accepted it. He laid the cookies on the front seat of his car, and the temptation to eat them was overpowering, so he called me.

That day, he just needed to be reassured that it would be okay to stop by the nearest dumpster and toss those cookies into it, even though they were a gift from well-meaning friends. And I told him that it would be perfectly fine to pitch them.

So he did.

Likewise, if you're at a crossroads and struggling with indecision, overwhelming temptations, and need reassurance...I am telling you that it is perfectly acceptable to toss whatever self-destructive food is tempting you. In fact, you must get rid of it if you want to escape being addicted to it. You'll have absolutely no regrets because living in freedom is like winning the lottery—only better, because it is a priceless treasure that enables you to enjoy life to the fullest!

It goes without saying that I hate what the toxic American diet has done to me, my family, and so many of you. The typical diet not only robs health, vitality, and finances, but relationships as well. When you're sluggish and barely functioning, relationships suffer, not to mention loss of life due to premature death for some.

It's time for all of us to put the shame and stigma of the "battle of the bulge" aside and band together to swim upstream against the powerful current of the Standard American Diet. We are not only fighting for our own health and well-being, but also for our children—and their children's future health. The current food culture wants us to succumb to the temptations that abound because it financially profits from our addictions.

Let's help each other blaze new trails, and, together, fight our way to victory!

It has been my honor and privilege to share this book with you, and I want to continue this conversation in the months and years to come. Plus, I'm sure that long after these words are in print, I will think of a kazillion other things to include.

I invite you to contact me at www.EmilyBoller.com or follow me on Facebook (Emily Boller "Starved to Obesity") or Instagram (emilysboller) in order to continue this conversation and stay in touch. I can't promise I'll reply to every message, but I will certainly do my best to read them and then respond to your comments. After all, we are on this journey together.

Also, if this book has resonated with you, and you feel stirred to spread this message, please consider writing a review on Amazon. Thank you very much.

Peace to you always.
Sincerely,
Emily

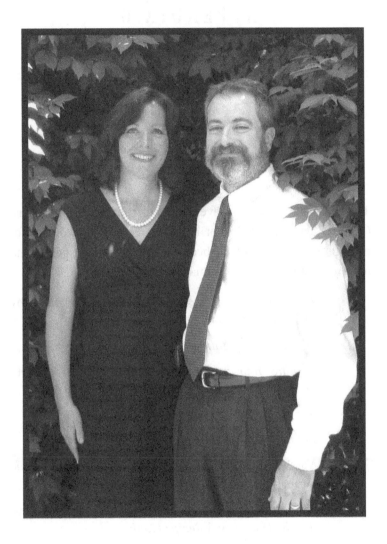

The End

APPENDIX D

HELPFUL RESOURCES

The following resources have helped me throughout these past (almost) ten years. I do not receive a commission or fee for recommending them. I have been blessed by these resources and merely want to pass the information along:

- *Toxic Churches: Restoration from Spiritual Abuse* by Marc Dupont

- *Understanding Your Grief* by Alan Wolfelt, Ph.D.

- *Healing Your Traumatized Heart* by Alan Wolfelt, Ph.D.

- *Eat to Live* by Joel Fuhrman, M.D.

- *Eat to Live Cookbook* by Joel Fuhrman, M.D.

- *Nutritarian Handbook and ANDI Food Scoring Guide* by Joel Fuhrman, M.D.

- Dr. Fuhrman's Member Center: *Nutritarian Network, Ask the Doctor,* and *Recipe Guide*

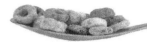

- Dr. Fuhrman's article: "Get Rid of the Winter Blues and Depression the Natural Way" (located in the library section of www.DrFuhrman.com)

- "The Compassionate Friends"; support for bereaved families after the death of a child
  - Seven hundred chapters worldwide with locations in all fifty states—www.compassionatefriends.org

- Healing Room Ministries–prayer support–www.HealingRooms.com

- www.Hope4MentalHealth.com; excellent resources for navigating mental health issues

- *The Rest Liturgy* by Andrew Booth; calming instrumental music (primarily flute)

ACKNOWLEDGMENTS

My heartfelt gratitude and thanks to:

Kurt, my husband of more than thirty-seven years, for his steadfast love and commitment to me and our marriage—and, along with our children—for riding the rollercoaster of food addiction with me, even though none of them signed up for it. I am forever grateful for their unconditional love and support shown to me.

Dr. Joel Fuhrman for his sacrificial and persevering commitment to discover the ongoing keys to optimal health; and for his genuine goodwill and care for the well-being of mankind. I am also grateful to him for believing in me and urging me to keep writing when the troll was on the loose—and for encouraging and mentoring my writing and speaking endeavors. I write and speak today, in part, because of him.

Dr. Carl Sovine for his wise counsel to Kurt and me throughout the past two decades. There are no words to adequately express the value of what he has done for our marriage except to quote King Solomon: "Counsel in the heart of man is like deep water; but a man of understanding will draw it out." (Proverbs 20:5, King James Version)

I am incredibly grateful to Dr. Jeffrey Rediger for offering his encouragement and professional expertise from the field of psychiatry; and to Dr. David Friedman, Dr. Scott Stoll, Dr.

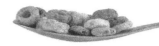

Michael Klaper, Dr. Rudy Kachmann, the Rev. Dr. Susan Gilbert Zencka, Ken Hood, Sarah Taylor, Kristen Meier, and Carol Doscher for taking the time from their busy schedules to offer their support as well.

I am also grateful to everyone who has helped bring this book to fruition: my son-in-law Zach Andrews for encouraging me to write again; my daughter Ruth Yaroslaski for shooting the images for the cover; Bradley Communications for casting vision and making connections; Deb Englander for patiently guiding me through each step of the publishing process; and special thanks to Post Hill Press for believing in the importance of championing this message to the world.

My sincerest gratitude goes to the following individuals who have profoundly influenced me in becoming the person that I am today:

- My parents, Robert and Helen Taylor, for rearing me in the nurture and admonition of the Lord.

- My Aunt Tee for always being there to cheer me on throughout my life.

- Al Pounders, professor emeritus of painting at Purdue University, for imparting a passion and desire to produce significant works of art.

- Mrs. Laurel Steill, my high school English teacher, for igniting a love of writing.

- Charles Shepard III, president and CEO of the Fort Wayne Museum of Art, and Kelly Kolterman, for their support of my art exhibit.

❧ Marc and Kim Dupont for moving to Fort Wayne when they did…and for inviting me to Singing Waters.

❧ My precious friends: Audrey Riley for her faithful support, laughter, and honesty through the crazy rollercoaster ride of the past decade; Angie Klarke for her steadfast prayers through the hard times; Sarah Taylor for always believing in me and encouraging me even when I had lost my way; Heidi Choi for going out of her way to cheer me on; and Claudia Dozier, Colleen Obergfell, Jackie Carsten, and Jackie Trainer for their friendship, prayers, and encouragement throughout the years.

❧ Dan and Tammy Rodgers; Ed, Pat, Doug, Cindy, and Jeanne Taylor; Ben and Lisa Boller; Bruce and Kristie Arnn; John and Pat Alexander; Don and Nancy Williams; Jeff and Sharon Hoffman; Max and Dolly Eleiott; Julie Thomas; Carl Marcum and family; the Women's Ministry at First Assembly Fort Wayne; Daisy Bailey; Vera Button; Linda Landrigan; Patsy Kauffman; Lois Smith; Stacia Alexander; Rhonda Kachmann; Linda Burd; Rebecca Justice Schaab; and Helen Haskell for their generosity and help in the midst of crisis.

❧ Pastor Ron Hawkins for gently shepherding me through trauma and recovery; and the many folks at First Assembly Fort Wayne, for praying for me through the dark valley to the other side.

❧ Bonnie Davis, MSW, LSW; Sharon Brockhaus, Ruby Hahn, Julie Brommer, and "The Compassionate Friends" for their gracious support through grief.

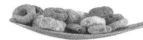

❧ My "battle buddies" in my small group family: Dave, Heidi, Greg, Maylynne, Kevin, Lori, and Robert for their love, prayers, and support.

❧ Dr. Fuhrman's Member Center for cheering me onward throughout the past decade. Your ongoing encouragement has been—and always will be—priceless to me.

❧ Above all, I am most grateful to God Almighty for being my ever-present help in times of trouble.

Soli Deo Gloria

ABOUT THE AUTHOR

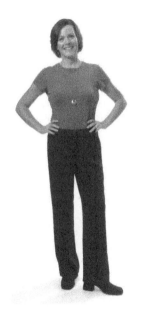

Emily Boller earned a Bachelor of Arts with Distinction in Fine Arts from Purdue University and certificates in Basic Nutrition and The Science of the Nutritarian Diet from the Nutritarian Education Institute.

Emily and her husband, Kurt, have been married for thirty-seven years, and together they have raised five children in the heart of the Midwest. She understands the challenges of healthy living in a culture bent on eating addictive and disease-causing food. After losing a child to suicide, she also knows the impact of trauma and grief on food addiction recovery as well. Besides writing and speaking, Emily is an artist who works primarily in the mediums of oil and watercolor paintings.

For more information, please visit www.EmilyBoller.com.